The MYTH of AUTISM

How a Misunderstood Epidemic
Is Destroying Our Children

Dr. Michael J. Goldberg
with Elyse Goldberg

Foreword by Dr. Ismael Mena

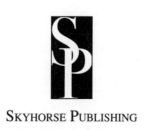

SKYHORSE PUBLISHING

www.skyhorsepublishing.com

10 9 8 7 6 5 4 3 2 1

Library of Congress Cataloging-in-Publication Data available on file.

ISBN: 978-1-61608-171-3

Printed in the United States of America

CONTENTS

Although the focus of this book is the autism myth, a lot of the information, studies, and conclusions can be applied to how we understand and approach ADHD variants, CFS, and CFIDS in children and adults (and to many other nonspecific psychiatric and learning labels applied to many "special needs" children today).

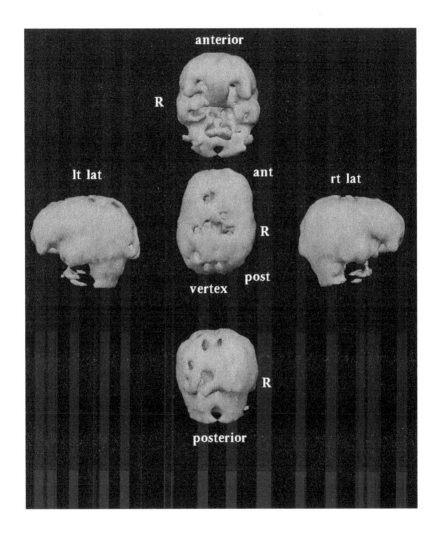

Initial 3-D NeuroSPECT imaging on patient with autism (see appendix A). "Holes" are multiple areas of decreased perfusion and decreased function in the brain. This brain scan graphically illustrates the difficulty of normal brain function when "holes" are present.

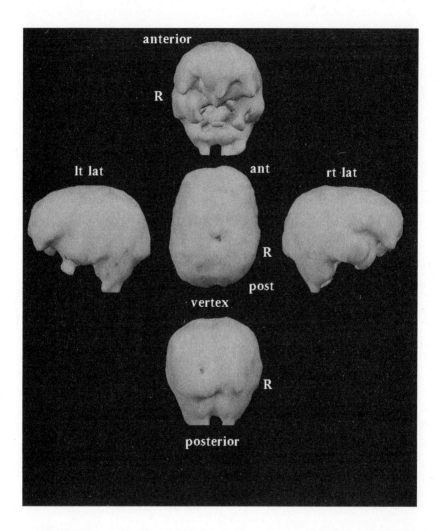

NeuroSPECT scan 2.5 years later, after treatment with The Goldberg Approach (see chapter 7). While brain function is not normal, it is significantly improved.

Conclusion: this disorder and its complications can be changed.

FOREWORD

Since 1994, Dr. Michael Goldberg and I have collaborated during my tenure as Director of the Department of Nuclear Medicine at Harbor-UCLA Medical Center in Torrance, California. The development of quantitative functional imaging techniques at our laboratory was instrumental for a long-standing collaboration in the challenging field of autism that Dr. Goldberg suspected from very early to be the consequence of an inflammatory process and thus amenable for treatment. Over the years, the epidemic increase of the prevalence of this dreadful condition has strengthened this hypothesis.

During the last fifteen years we have participated actively in the development of quantitative software in order to assess brain perfusion by means of NeuroSPECT. The development of this imaging software has achieved results by comparing against a normal, age-matched database and expressed in standard deviations above or below the normal mean. (The color gray is normal range, whereas light blue, dark blue, and green denote hypoperfusion at 2, 3, and 4 standard deviations below the normal, age-matched mean, respectively. The colors red, pink, and white are 2, 3, and 4 standard deviations above normal mean, respectively). The process entails normalization of brain volume in order to establish the comparisons mentioned above, and this is achieved by means of the Talairach technique, which is currently performed by automatic reconstruction, thus reaching the ultimate goal of 100 percent reproducibility of results (Segami Corp. Neurogam Oasis). This highly accurate way of assessing brain perfusion, and therefore of brain function, is performed with the radiopharmaceutical Tc^{99m} HMPAO, Ceretec, that provides stability of distribution and concentration in the brain parenchyma after the first two minutes of IV injection with a 1 percent / hour loss only.

The NeuroSPECT findings of cerebral cortical and subcortical perfusion in chronic fatigue syndrome (CFS) and in pervasive developmental disorders, namely, autism, have enabled us to define common features among these two disorders. [1, 2, 3, 4] I've included these findings, in brief, to give the reader a sense of the extensive research that informs *The Myth of Autism*.

Chronic Fatigue Syndrome

Patients with CFS present during the evolution of their chronic condition signs of small vessel disease distributed in the lateral aspects of temporal lobes, premotor areas, and parietal lobes reaching to the convexity of the brain and also in the orbital-frontal areas of the frontal lobes. There is also frequent involvement of temporal lobes in the mesial aspects, in the projection of the hippocampus, and in the inferior gyrus at the level of the temporal poles also. In the limbic system we observe diminished function in anterior and posterior cingulate gyri and approximately in 50 percent of patients hypoperfusion in the subgenual area thus implying the presence of a secondary depression. Finally there is focal hypoperfusion also in both occipital lobes in the interhemispheric fissure, highlighted in this patient in the posterior view and inferior aspects of temporal and occipital lobes. In the subcortical structures there is very frequently deep hypoperfusion of the head of the caudate nuclei, less frequently in the dorso-ventral posterior aspects of both thalami and some times also hypoperfusion in the lentiform nuclei. The findings of subgenual hypoperfusion, anterior cingulate hypoperfusion, and increased thalamic perfusion are indicative of the presence secondary depression. The caudate and posterior cingulate gyrus hypoperfusion in the presence of hippocampus hypoperfusion are indicative in other patients of cognitive dysfunction, which is a frequent symptom in CFS. These findings suggest severe inflammatory changes involving, temporal, frontal, parietal lobes, occipital lobes, and frequently caudate nuclei involvement denoting cognitive impairment.

Autism

Quantitative rCBF absolute measurements with Xenon 133 were found to be significantly higher than normal in autistic children, with maximal values in the frontal lobes and visual cortex. Minimal perfusion was observed in the temporal lobes. Decreased rCBF was also noted in the cerebellum and occipital lobe. Tc 99m HMPAO images demonstrate qualitatively increased frontal (subgenual) perfusion, and also temporal, occipital hypoperfusion. In this patient increased subgenual perfusion is indicative of a comorbidity of attention deficit disorder.

In other patients we have demonstrated with Tc 99m HMPAO imaging increased frontal perfusion, and also temporal, occipital, and cerebellar hypoperfusion. In the basal ganglia of these patients very frequently there is normal perfusion and function of thalami, caudate nuclei, and lentiform nuclei. They may also have many symptoms consistent with OCD characteristics, associated with the following areas of dysfunction, namely, inferior frontal, anterior poles of the temporal lobes (amygdala), and posterior cingulate gyri, demonstrating increased perfusion of these areas.

In 1995, Mountz, Tolbert, Lill, Katholi, and Liu reported their HMPAO findings in six children with severe autism and demonstrated with semiquantitative techniques temporal and parietal hypoperfusion with lateralization to the left hemisphere.

Georges, Costa, Coniz, Ring, and Ell reported in four autistic adults with Tc-99 HMPAO diminished rCBF in temporal and frontal lobes. The temporal abnormality appears to be confirmed mostly in adults, adolescents, and children suffering of autism. Thus, damage to temporal lobe in an early developmental stage may result in autistic manifestations.

The results are otherwise heterogeneous, denoting the presence of occipital hypoperfusion and cerebellar hypoperfusion mostly in the mesial aspects corresponding to the vermis area. This later observation correlates with reports in the literature of atrophy of the cerebellar vermis demonstrated by MRI technique. Further heterogeneity in our group of patients is demonstrated by apparent comorbidity with OCD and ADHD in these children and their typical presentation of increased perfusion in lateral frontal lobes.

In Asperger's syndrome the hypoperfusion defects appear predominantly in occipital lobes in the paramedial aspects and also in the cerebellar vermis.

In both chronic fatigue syndrome and autism the multifocal areas described—strikingly in the occipital lobes and always more extensively in temporal lobes—suggest strongly the inflammatory nature of both disorders, at vascular or cellular level (vasculatis versus cellular damage), thus opening expectations for early diagnosis and hopefully for treatment for these and other potentially related crippling diseases.

Ismael Mena, MD

Emeritus Professor Radiological Sciences
UCLA School of Medicine

Doctor Honoris Causa
University d'Auvergne, France

Department of Nuclear Medicine
Clinica Las Condes
Santiago, Chile

INTRODUCTION

WHEN I GRADUATED FROM UCLA MEDICAL School as a pediatrician in 1972, I was told if I had even one autistic child in my practice it would be unusual. Today most of my practice (250–300 active patients at any time) is composed of children and young adults diagnosed on the autistic spectrum, something we were never prepared for in medical school. General pediatrician practices now have between six and twelve children on the spectrum or with significant learning difficulties. I have heard from parents that their pediatricians were as unprepared as I was for this onslaught. So how is it that in thirty years the rate of "autism" in American children has gone from nonexistent to affecting nearly 1 percent of the total population or even higher?

To understand this change, let me give you some history. After I failed handwriting in the third grade, my teacher joked that I should become a doctor. Growing up, I enjoyed math and science, liked working with people and children, and did not envision myself in a lab with test tubes, so medicine, and in particular pediatrics, became my goal. I was extremely thankful to be accepted into UCLA Medical School, and I remain thankful for the wonderful training, for my internship and residency in pediatrics spent at Los Angeles County–University of Southern California Medical Center, with rotations through Children's Hospital of Los Angeles. What I learned within these institutions gave me an excellent background in infectious disease, immunology, allergies, and more. The professors and the medical system to which I was exposed formed a dynamic, exciting system. There was still the expectation that a physician would use a combination of clinical skills and emerging technologies to help advance their understanding and take their research to new levels. Medicine was viewed as a frontier that needed to be consistently explored. This expectation was quickly dropped when it came to researching the causes of a rising disease called autism.

I entered private practice in Tarzana, California, with optimism and excitement. I built the third largest pediatric practice in the San Fernando Valley in Los Angeles. On a busy day, I could see up to fifty-two children. I would never let a sick child wait for an appointment if it were at all possible. I was taught preventive medicine in medical school; I was a good pediatrician if few children needed admittance to the hospital. The United States has evolved rapidly to a system where hospitals encourage admissions, however. Sadly, our collective "health" now boils down to dollars and cents.

Back then, for example, the standard practice was to postpone immunization for a child if he or she had a cold or a fever; parents would bring the child back for the shots once he or she was healthy. Economics now dictates that we limit visits. The more we bill at one time, the better, so let's vaccinate them with everything we can give them while they are here in the office, all in the name of efficiency.

What new vaccines are being added to the roster of necessary childhood vaccinations, and why? How many readers are aware that the fairly recent decision by the Academy of Pediatrics in 1991 to give a hepatitis B vaccine in the newborn nursery[1] (the most dangerous adjustment time in a baby's life) was not made on the rational basis of medical efficacy but, in large part, due to the sticky issue of political correctness? It would not be PC to point out the limited number of cases where a child *might* be returning to a high-risk home, so let's vaccinate *all* the infants. (For the record, I never have given that shot in the nursery, and many pediatricians now have no problem if parents elect to defer that vaccination until later.)

In the early eighties I met the woman who would become my wife. Around fifteen months after we met, Elyse developed a mysterious illness that at that time had no name—she was suffering sudden severe headaches, overwhelming fatigue, constant short-term memory issues and often periods of severe brain fog, fibromyalgia muscle and joint symptoms, fevers, and swollen glands. She visited various doctors all around the country, but she remained miserable and undiagnosed. Her blood work came back positive for an astounding number of viruses—almost every virus she was tested for excluding HIV. While she tested positive for Epstein-Barr, CMV (cytomegalovirus), HHV6, rubeola, and rubella, to name a few, it was rapidly obvious that while some of these titers might represent a potential virus to target, others were just false activation from a dysfunctional or misdirected (perhaps an unidentified virus or retrovirus) immune system. With these test results in hand, it seemed logical to suspect that some of these viruses (not as a new acute infection, but with the new concept of reactivation) were causing an impairment of her immune system or that somehow her immune system was making mistakes. Healthy patients do not run around with three or four active viruses in their bodies, or even multiple elevated titers—although some of the medical profession didn't see any significance to the results of these blood tests, whether true viruses or just false titers, there was no direct evidence as far as they were concerned that this was causing harm (retrospectively this was a very large mistake).

She was sick and scared. As a physician I felt helpless, and we turned to prescription-grade vitamins and amino acids, thinking maybe they would help address any imbalances in her system. She took sixty-eight supplements a day, leaving little room for food with all the liquid she needed to swallow them. It was years before she would have a diagnosis. It is both sad and ironic that some of the same treatments tried on her then and others we never would have allowed (because they were potentially harmful) are being used on children today with about the same success rate of close to nothing. Of more concern is preliminary evidence (with formal study being planned) from NeuroSPECT testing showing potential increased stress to children's brains when they undergo some of the more untested treatment ideas (including chelation, hyperbaric oxygen, and megasupplements).

We were married, and her symptoms continued. One night at dinner my son, around four years old at the time, said, "Dad, why are you sending Mom all over the country? Why don't you just fix her?" This began my journey into the complex workings of the neuroimmune system and how it controls the body and our brains.

1

IN THE BEGINNING

I N THE EARLY EIGHTIES, I WAS starting to see a shift in the concerns of the patients in my practice. Children were tired. Moms started complaining they couldn't keep up or that they were feeling "spacey" or "zoney." This was troubling, since early in my career I could safely joke that if a mother checked the fine print on her child's birth certificate, she was not allowed to get sick until the child was at least eighteen years old. I had to stop saying that, since mothers were among the first being hit by what was facetiously being called the "yuppie flu." Running viral blood titers (measurement of specific viral antibodies in their bloodstream/serum) on these patients was eye-opening. We were taught in medical school you were only supposed to have one active virus at a time, and "old" titers were supposed to be present but at low numbers. These patients were presenting with multiple viruses evident. A theory evolved that the immune system was so dysfunctional, it mistakenly thought it was fighting many viruses. How could so many moms and children be walking around and functioning with obvious evidence for some type of a severe autoimmune or viral disorder going on? After a few years, I attended the First International Congress on Chronic Fatigue in 1990 hosted by Dr. Jay Goldstein, who was beginning to define this new illness that had been given the official (but deliberately demeaning) name of Chronic Fatigue Syndrome by the Centers for Disease Control two years earlier in 1988. Dr. Goldstein and other clinicians were using the term postviral fatigue syndrome/chronic fatigue syndrome (the British still use the term ME—myalgic encephalomyelitis). The CDC made the official criteria/definition in 1988. Several years later, I had the honor of cohosting, and our journey toward understanding began in earnest. At these conferences I met many great doctors, including Dr. Nancy Klimas, who would finally offer some answers. Dr. Klimas sat my wife down and explained the immune system to her. She explained how it worked and, if you pushed the wrong buttons, how it didn't.

Those sixty-eight amino acids my wife was taking were from a company that at the time was producing amino acids of pharmaceutical grade (which in theory could be absorbed safely by the body). Since amino acids are the basic building blocks of proteins and other biomolecules, and play a role in energy pathways, it was a good premise: the company would take a patient's blood specimen, analyze it, and then decide what mixture of supplements (proportion of amino acids and some vitamins) you needed to take to help the body get back to normal. In medical school, and in a summer internship, I was fortunate to study under Dr. Ben Kagan (Cedars-Sinai Hospital–UCLA). Several years, before he passed away, I got the courage to ask him about supplements. I was particularly interested in lysine, a key essential amino acid, for its known ability to fight viruses—and I thought the strange viruses in my wife's blood might be cured with the proper amino acid treatments. "What do you think about amino acid supplements?" Ben looked at me, and he said, "You know, Michael, we tried to do that—help make a child healthier with amino acid supplements—but the first problem was that you have to have the proper ratio of arginine [the other key amino acid tied with the immune system, but a problem since it could strengthen, feed herpes-related viruses] to lysine. But way more important, we couldn't get it past the liver." I was told that this research had already been done in Boston back in the 1930s, and it had also been unsuccessful because they could not get the amino acids through the liver. Because the animo acids could not be absorbed, it was impossible to strengthen the right pathways in the body through supplementation. The medical community acknowledged that the concept had potential, but it seemed impractical. Dr. Kagan told me that most OTC (over-the-counter) products would not work because they could never be absorbed by the human body or pass the blood-brain barrier. Our bodies are designed to protect us from foreign substances—that's why the acid in our stomachs is so strong and why we have a liver, other filtering devices, and protective cells.

Back at my practice, investigating if this avenue of therapy could really help, I was doing a lot of amino acid profiles. This test measured serum amino acid levels, in the belief that the "pattern" was predictive of the type of disease and some of the dysfunctions that were occurring, and in theory a guide on how to try to help change that by supporting the body in a very directed nutritional manner. I was noticing a similar pattern in both the children and the adults I was testing. By this time, I had begun to treat some of the parents of the children in my practice who were complaining of this generalized, nonspecific illness.

My practice began to grow, but instead of seeing newborns for wellness checkups, I was seeing chronic fatigue patients and children with CFS and children with mixed attention deficit and hyperactivity disorder (ADHD) and quiet attention deficit disorder (ADD) that we had never been taught about in medical school (because these categories had not existed at that time). One of my colleagues whose practice had yet to see a similar increase in these types of complaints joked that it must only be happening on my side of the street. How I wish that statement had been true.

While I was working with these amino acid profiles, using the company's research and testing, looking at applications of their recommendations in products, the company sent me files of a group of families from West Los Angeles who had children with autism. Their head researcher had noted an early similarity in their testing and that of adults with chronic fatigue syndrome. They wanted me to run additional amino acid profiles, viral titers, and also candida (a form of yeast) titers on these children. At that time, you were considered a borderline quack if you even said the word *candida*. If I said I believed yeast caused the dysfunction in these children or adults, researchers I respect and counted on would have never spoken with me again, because I would have been a fool. If I qualified my discussion, noted that work on adults had confirmed that when the immune system is stressed, what we call "delayed hypersensitivity" is off or dysfunctional, the issue was open for discussion. At that point, anyone, a child or adult, is prone to a potential yeast or fungal overgrowth. Unless critically ill, this overgrowth will be appropriately restricted to the GI tract (sometimes vaginal area in females), sometimes the skin externally, but will not be found in a patient's blood, their brain, or any other primary internal organ. In that way, yeast or candida can be a symptom—evidence of the stress on the body—but not the reason or cause. When I ran these tests, I made an interesting discovery. I noticed that the results of the amino acid profiles for the children with autism were similar to the results of these adults and other children whom I was seeing and treating in my practice for these generalized symptoms of chronic fatigue syndrome and the new ADHD variants. When one realizes that a previously high-functioning, type A, college-trained "yuppie" does not know why they went to the kitchen or drove to the end of the block, cannot remember the right word to say, and becomes overwhelmed in loud places and prone to panic attacks and anxiety attacks, one gains a tremendous insight as to what is really happening to these children, how bad they must feel, how terrified they must be at times, when we are completely misinterpreting them. I ran immune panels, viral titers, ANAs (antinuclear antibodies), and did NeuroSPECTs (brain Single Photon Emission Computed Tomography— an imaging technique showing blood flow in the brain using a low-dose radiologic isotope, with the rationale that blood flow correlates directly and objectively to brain function). There was an overlap of patterns of multiple viral titer elevations to Epstein-Barr, CMV (cytomegalovirus) and HHV6 (human herpes virus 6), and low NK cells (frequently below 4 or 5 percent—a key marker for immune dysfunction in children and adults). On NeuroSPECT the "autistic" children's brains showed abnormalities nearly identical to those of the adults and older children in my practice—that is, a temporal lobe hypoprofusion affecting their function and specifically areas of memory, social skills, auditory processing, and language—all the deficits we mistakenly blame on autism. The results floored me. "What does autism have to do with the immune system?" I wondered. I, like everybody else at that time, had not even begun to consider the fact that the symptoms of "autism" might be caused by an illness. At that time, autism was considered to be a mysterious disorder with no known cause. Since patients seemed "psychotic," and it was an era of psychiatry deeply set in Freudian theories ("refrigerator parenting" was thought to be a key reason for this psychological disorder), autism was defined as a form of childhood schizophrenia. The key point is when Dr. Kanner himself was asked what separated a child with this new idea of autism from classic childhood schizophrenia, Dr. Kanner's response was, "The child with autism was never affectionate." Based on that statement alone, 99.9 percent of the children today would not have "autism," and the medical world would really have to be trying to figure out what was happening to these children. Without the myth of autism, we would be figuring out how a disease process could strike down and destroy a potentially normal child— not children mysteriously miswired, congenitally beyond hope of a true recovery (the basis for the concepts we call "autism").

When Elyse realized these children had similar viral titers and immune markers as she had, she looked at me almost in tears and said, "If these children feel even one-tenth as bad as I did, you *have* to do something!" As an adult, although she hadn't understood what was happening to her body, she had at least known she wasn't normal. But these were children. "Mike," she implored, "they don't know what 'well' feels like. They have no basis for comparison. They may not know their brains don't work. They believe this is all there is. There can't be much quality of life." She wanted me to take action.

But where to begin?

After approximately seven years of research and eighteen months of my treating Elyse with very primitive immune modulators and whatever else I could get my hands on to improve her immune system, (with the knowledge that there was no conclusive evidence that these agents were helpful, I would meticulously avoid any agent that we knew in theory could be potentially harmful to a normal, physiologic brain or body; I follow this strict policy to this day, and it has served me well), my wife returned to function and, as she puts it, "the world." It is hard to believe looking back just how dysfunctional she was. Elyse has a very high IQ and graduated from college at nineteen years of age; she was not used to forgetting why she walked into the kitchen or where she left her keys, not experiencing "forgetfulness" (as can happen to anyone) but periods of brain fog, making it impossible to think. Short-term memory loss was a constant issue. One day she told me she felt as if a switch in her body had been turned on, and she felt well and continued to do better. Elyse jokes that she doesn't remember getting married; the countless vacations we took with the children (two girls from my previous marriage and a boy from her previous marriage) are hard for her to recall. Thank goodness for pictures! It is a travesty that the expanding idea of "autism spectrum disorder" has become a wastebasket diagnosis and an excuse for the medical community to abandon research, treatments, and hope for so many ill patients. At my first talk at the Autism Society of America my wife elbowed me and asked, "Where are the doctors?" While I was a medical doctor and keynote speaker, most of the other speakers were PhDs, and the audience mostly parents. While I was presenting NeuroSPECT scans of the brain, actual pictures of what was going on in the brain of sick children, and offering a medical reason for the dysfunction—a possible disease process, not a developmental disorder—it didn't seem to matter beyond the walls of the conference! If the medical profession does not address this as a problem to be solved, how will parents and thousands of affected children ever hope for an answer? Children are showing classic symptoms of viral disorders, true encephalopathies, yet these symptoms are ignored because these children are labeled autistic. It is beyond rational.

As a physician, I understand that the previous ideas of developmental learning difficulties (i.e., autism, ADHD, childhood dementias), which were once under the guidance and the control of psychiatry, should be no longer viable. Pediatricians and parents are being faced with a rapidly enlarging medical epidemic. The starting point of research, the starting focus needs to be that of figuring out a true medical epidemic, not of disproving a nonobjective, psychiatry-based "label." Without this change in focus, years more will be wasted and millions of dollars will continue to be misdirected to nonproductive ends.

So where did it all begin?

In Dr. Leo Kanner's now-classic 1943 research paper, he outlined the behavior pattern, present from early in life, that he named "early infantile autism." Prior to this, there were, in the literature, occasional accounts of individual children whose behavior fit the picture Kanner later described. Kanner described only the autistic children referred to his clinic and, later on, those attending a particular special school (Kanner, 1955). He made no estimates of the numbers in the general population, but he thought that this syndrome was rare.

Later, Kanner and Eisenberg (1956) discussed Kanner's original conception of autism and the five features he considered to be diagnostic. These were a profound lack of affective contact with other people; an anxiously obsessive desire for the preservation of sameness in the child's routines and environment; a fascination for objects, which are handled with skill in fine motor movements (an area of actual weakness in many of the children being diagnosed today); mutism or a kind of language that does not seem intended for interpersonal communication; and good cognitive potential shown in feats of memory or skills on performance tests, especially the Séguin form board. Kanner also emphasized onset from birth or before thirty months.

In the same paper, Kanner and Eisenberg modified the diagnostic criteria by selecting two as essential.

These were

1. a profound lack of affective contact and
2. repetitive, ritualistic behavior, which must be of an elaborate kind.

They considered that, if these two features were present, the rest of the typical clinical picture would also be found.

Rates of autism in 1956: 1 child in 10,000.

Rates of autism in 2011: with 1 child in 110 now the official CDC number, most current discussions are using 1 child in 91, with much higher numbers being quoted routinely (1:80 in the military!).

So, how can so many children now have such a previously rare disorder? How can a rare, almost unheard-of "severe mental dysfunction" become something every pediatrician is seeing, something every parent is concerned about? How can we now have this rare misfortune threaten to overwhelm our school and social systems while destroying families across this country and around the world?

To understand this, one needs to go back to the beginning. Per above, Kanner (1943) described a disorder according to its "behavioral" features. Needless to say, "behavioral" dysfunction can be caused by many factors, *not* just the idea of a developmental or psychiatric dysfunction.

Think of it: a general idea noting patterns of behavior held to be true over decades, with *only* a "behavioral" pattern for diagnosis, not one objective or consistent physiologic dysfunction or finding required to prove or disprove this "disorder/diagnosis" (but somehow all these children have it for life). Health professionals have no idea what causes this disorder. Explanations have ranged from childhood schizophrenia to bad parenting to something biologic, all with the underlying concept that "something" must have happened developmentally. Somehow (mechanism unknown) the brain was miswired; these children were not okay, could not be okay (but with no idea of what was happening, or why or how it happened).

> If one goes back and reviews the literature of the 1940s and 1950s, there was no support for or even a discussion of a genetic linkage. I have proposed there is no more evidence of a genetic connection today than the now fully disputed, insulting idea of a "refrigerator mom."

In the world I trained in, a rapid increase of affected children all showing a similar pattern of behavior should have created appropriate questions and initiated scientific, medical investigations. What's going on? Why are we suddenly seeing so many dysfunctional children? Maybe something is wrong here? Maybe this is not autism? The initial diagnosis has just kept expanding and modifying, and all the new children are just being put into a variation of the old basket. Instead of expanding the alphabet soup of autism (PDD, Asperger's, autistic spectrum, LKS [Landau-Kleffner syndrome], etc.), or likewise ADD (from a hyper, usually intelligent child, we evolved new labels for the different children appearing as mixed ADHD, quiet ADHD, ADD without hyperactivity, and many more), perhaps experts could have said maybe this is not just something we can label autism; maybe this is not the ADHD we were trained to treat. Maybe we have another problem (with some "autistic" or ADHD-like symptoms) occurring. Maybe we need to ask the critical questions: Do these children even fit this label? How many parents (often against their own belief) presently are being told their children have this strange disorder called "autism" (or are on the spectrum) and they must learn to live with it, accept it? How many parents think their children even come close to meeting Kanner's main criteria: "a *profound* lack of affective contact and elaborate repetitive, ritualistic behavior"? Kanner made a very important distinction, one that perhaps we should all be applying now. He separated a child with this new idea of autism from the child with childhood schizophrenia. Remember that it was all a psychiatric disease; Dr. Kanner's statement was that a child with autism was "never affectionate." Now if all we do is apply that one criteria (as we've applied the ritualistic behavior criteria exclusively today), 99.99 percent of these children would be classified with an illness, and not as having autism, and that would certainly become a pathway to a more desirable outcome than what we have now.

The precedent is that there has never been an epidemic of any type of genetic or developmental disorder. There are no exceptions. And yet, the vast majority of the researchers in this country, and throughout the world, are still studying these children as if they had some undefined, unknown "developmental" disorder. Instead of focusing on what can be understood only as a disease (not developmental) process, the system continues to fund researchers trying to figure out and understand "autism" (as a developmental disorder), and an ever-expanding list of connected physical problems.

This is why so little progress has occurred in spite of millions of dollars being spent. Researchers are being funded to study what the vast majority of the children appearing today cannot have. If this process continues, everyone will lose (except the researchers and universities receiving mass amounts of funding as well as the industry of alternative therapists helping to try and treat these "special needs" children).

It is blatantly obvious that 99.99 percent of affected children do not come close to meeting Kanner's definition of autism. The overwhelming majority of children being diagnosed as "autistic" do not have autism (as the term is understood or used), but rather are exhibiting symptoms of a disease state, a CNS (central nervous system) dysfunction. This dysfunction resembles a true medical encephalopathy, rather than anything called "autism". Unlike a developmental disorder, this disease is treatable if we act quickly enough. How many of the the existing autism groups are questioning present funding, present efforts? How many are going before Congress protesting that we have a large group of children that if helped, if treated, might grow up to be productive citizens, might pay taxes (rather than requiring more and more social services) one day? Why *not*?

That is "the myth of autism." Children are being labeled with a disorder they do not really have. Parents are being told there is little hope, when there should be a lot of reasons for hope. As long as we continue to label so many children and families with this undefined, unexplained disorder, few physicians, parents, or politicians expect these children could ever recover or regain regular function. The myth of autism is perpetuating many dangerous or partially successful therapies, with some success (often with large risks) being better than nothing.

What bothers me is the autistic child who spends the day at a special school with five to ten other children and copies their bad behaviors rather than learning from a normal child.

What if physicians and therapists expected a child to recover and focused on finding answers to fix this now, for this generation of children, rather than accepting any degree of minute improvement as wonderful? What if we could bring the children and parents of this generation back to the field of pediatrics that existed when I trained?

It has become obvious that neuroimmune and/or chronic viral connections are the only possible cause, the only proposed mechanisms that have no scientific *contradictions* and an ever-enlarging compendium of articles *in support*. While many will pose the question "Where are the controlled studies?" every medical fact and recent discovery helps substantiate the likelihood of an autoimmune, neuroimmune-related process.

We are presently at a crossroads. Are we going to continue to blindly follow old logic, old thinking with no consistent physiologic dysfunction measurable or documented, or can we unite behind scientifically sound data, more than reasonable medical probability and clinical logic, before we lose forever the chance to help this generation of children? There are excellent researchers, clinicians, and scientists ready to focus on solving this disease now, rather than study the myth, but this effort to fight a disease (NIDS, or whatever name is eventually used) remains buried under the wall of controlled misinformation. This is now obviously a medical crisis, a true medical epidemic that should no longer be under the supervision of psychiatry, but should be relocated to the realm of pediatric infectious disease, pediatric immunology, and a medically focused pediatric neurology.

Unless we all step up now to change this, to demand clinical science and logic, not mythology, the system could easily take another ten to fifteen years (or longer) to come around to the right answers. How many are ready to step up and say, "Enough is enough"? How many millions of dollars have been spent (particularly in the last six to seven years) with no answers and without any new hope?

The NIDS effort was formed to help look at this crisis appropriately, scientifically, logically, and medically. Many parents are working hard to help make a real future for their children. (Visit their site @ www.NIDS.net.)

At an NIH-sponsored conference many years ago (1996), presenting my preliminary NeuroSPECT work with Dr. Ismael Mena and Dr. Bruce Miller, before a room full of high-level researchers, including many Nobel laureates, I expressed cautiously (expecting resistance to this idea) that if this process hits you as an adult, you get CFS or the new idea of adult ADHD. If it hits you as a teenager or older child, you get ADD/ADHD variants or CFS/CFIDS. But if this process hits you as a young child, with an immature brain an immature immune system, you get autism/PDD. They did not laugh (or ban me from future conferences), and, two years later, at the next conference many were coming up to express their agreement. As that was 1998, it remains a sad mystery to me today why more money and more resources have not been allocated to a medical investigation of "autism."

It is my fervent hope that in the near future the existence of an immune dysfunctional/dysregulatory state will be commonly accepted, whether the patient exhibits fatigue or not. Perhaps we will come to recognize that an immune dysregulatory state is a generalized condition that may include many interrelated phenomena, such as CFS/CFIDS, atypical and/or typical rheumatoid disease, most if not nearly all of autism, and parts of ADHD, as well as other learning disabilities. It seems probable that this disease has an element of genetic predisposition (confirmed in emerging epidemiologic studies). In following a number of families in my practice, I have found that not all members of the same family become ill. Often one child and/or one parent alone is affected. This likely implies a lack of ongoing contagion, if any, associated with this syndrome, suggesting genetic predisposition with probable multiple triggering agents or events. These can include viruses, a combination of stresses, or various traumas, setting off a state in the body in which the immune system, the CNS, or both do not come back to a normal functioning level. As supported by many peer-reviewed papers, once this process is in motion it is controlled by the innate immune system, not the initiating stress or stressors (or any kind of a simple genetic chromosomal defect).

The social-educational-economic implications of all of this are terrifying. We are running out of money and bankrupting educational systems to deal with the epidemic of special-needs children. I have nothing but respect (and sympathy) for teachers, who are on the front lines, being asked to do their best to educate a growing number of affected children. With all the studies on all the possible reasons for this, how many have thought of looking at the bigger picture? These children are all points on a bell curve. Rather than just exhibiting multiple variants of learning difficulties, put under different labels, these children really are ill and have part of their brains not working. How much more successful would these teachers be, how much could we begin to dream of lowering education costs, at minimum being far more effective for all students, if we recognized that, as physicians and parents, we have an obligation to send children to school alert and healthy? Whatever the combination of factors, once in motion, there is likely a medically definable problem that can be treated. We must stop assuming these children's function is carved in stone, determined in some mysterious way genetically, developmentally.

I continue to believe awareness and recognition of the true medical crisis being discussed in this book will mean parents and children receive more help, but help focused and dedicated in the right direction. For, if helped, with children's body and brains made healthy, the system will not only smile at its success but also save hundreds of millions (at this point likely hundreds of billions) of dollars in now unneeded expenses.

2

HOW CAN THIS BE ANYTHING
BUT AN ILLNESS?

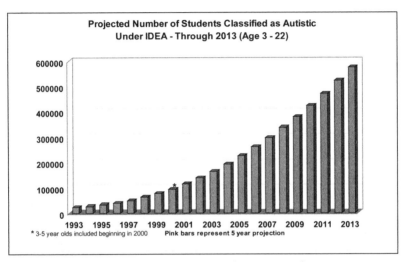

Graphs produced by Anthony E. Vizioli

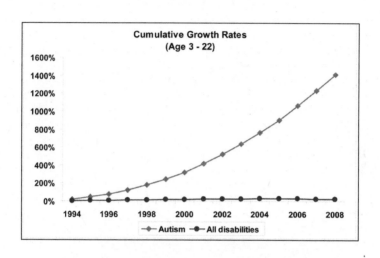

Cumulative Growth Rates
(Age 3 - 22)

— Autism — All disabilities

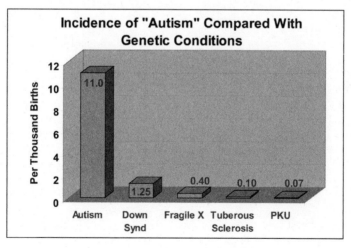

Incidence of "Autism" Compared With
Genetic Conditions

U NLIKE DOWN SYNDROME, FRAGILE X, AND other common childhood disorders that have a genetic link, can be evident at birth, and whose rates have remained stable in the last fifty years, autism rates are increasing rapidly across the globe, affecting childhood populations in numbers similar to medical epidemics of the past like the Spanish flu and the bubonic plague. This disease affects children after they are born. It is acquired, like other illnesses. Based on early clinical work and reports, linked by the emerging NeuroSPECT results (the use of a low-dose radioisotope and imaging to measure blood flow, which defines function in areas of the brain), I and a few other physicians coined the term NIDS (Neuro Immune Dysfunction Syndromes) as a way to try to create a *medical* umbrella over the previously *developmental* categories of ADHD, autism, and other now likely immune-medicated (a CNS system, neuroimmune-created dysfunction in key areas of the brain) learning or cognitive disorders. The NIDS hypothesis was first discussed in early 2000, and found wide agreement with no scientific debate or dispute by researchers and pharmaceutical representatives who read it. It just made sense.

Under the umbrella of NIDS, the multiple secondary metabolic, physiologic, and immune markers that are abnormal in these children make sense. The "new" family constellation presenting to many physicians begins to make sense. Representing nothing I was ever taught about in medical school, internship, or residency, there was now a newly emerging family constellation of a mother or father with CFS/CFIDS or "other" immune mediated disorder, an older child (or two) with an ADHD variant (or other learning disorder), and a younger child (or two) with autism or PDD. This pattern is impossible for a developmental or genetic disorder. It is the logical result of a complex neuroimmune, complex viral connection with NIDS.

Let's go back to the symptoms and forget the label. If we remove the diagnosis of autism and simply look at the symptoms, we see a variety of common factors. Typical medical histories include immune-related issues of eczema, hives, or other allergic issues, along with recurrent ear infections, frequent sore throats, and flulike illnesses.

Confusing for many parents and health professionals is the fact that many "normal" children will typically also experience recurrent infections, recurrent ear infections, a stressed delivery, and recurrent allergies and not fall into this complex disorder (NIDS). The logic is simple when one understands that most normal children in the past were not born under already-stressed circumstances (many adults and children now have activated immune systems compared to the normal baselines of four or five decades ago), and then depending upon the combination and number of stressors, while most of them will manage to recover and come back to an acceptable baseline; an enlarging group of infants and children are being pushed over the edge into this complex neuroimmune, then complex viral dysfunctional state. It is interesting that as with a "normal" child, some of these children, probably dependent upon their allergy responses, have a history of recurrent congestion and then recurrent infections, while some (usually those without the congestion issues or in whom the triggers for congestion have been removed) will generally seem to stay healthy and not present with recurrent ear, sinus, or chest infections. My overwhelming experience for years with a large "normal" pediatric practice (in which some children were prone to allergies) was in how to keep a child clear, and how to avoid recurrent congestion/infections.

Common symptoms of neurological dysfunction (rather than a psychologically based disorder) include trouble concentrating that can be described as "spacey" or "zoney;" a sensory, auditory, or vestibular processing difficulty; "executive dysfunction"; sleep difficulties or an abnormal sleep cycle; and fine or gross motor abnormalities. As noted elsewhere, these findings, particularly the fine and gross motor issues, become markers for the likelihood of a virus occurring. If one goes back to the autism literature of the 1940s and 1950s, there is no mention of fine or gross motor issues.

The presence of the above symptoms should demand a medical focus and a medical evaluation. We can no longer continue to ignore or discredit it. If we remove the label called autism and again focus on the patient, the child, we can begin to deal with symptoms that without the hysteria, without the misconceptions of "autism," would be regarded as a true medical crisis.

How We Got Here

Unfortunately, without the tools or the technology to accurately investigate the human brain, the label of autism evolved from the observation of a set of symptoms in a dysfunctional child. In its most severe form ("classic autism"), effective speech was absent, and clinicians often saw symptoms of repetitive, highly unusual aggressive and sometimes self-injurious behavior. Those afflicted had extremely abnormal ways of relating to people, objects, or events. Parents noticed that something was "not right," often within the first three to six months of life. These children typically did not smile and often resisted affection.

Most researchers and clinicians did not look for medical answers to autism (likewise ADD/ADHD and most childhood learning or psychological disorders) because they believed it was a disorder that was medically untreatable. Without the technology to understand these children, pediatricians and pediatric psychologists accepted the concepts of poor parenting or childhood psychosis/schizophrenia and classified autism as a psychological and/or developmental disorder. Psychologists and psychiatrists typically delivered treatment.

In accordance with this premise, recent discussions have focused on the difference between "congenital autism" (including "classic" Kanner autism) and another form related to neurologic and medical disorders such as tuberous sclerosis, phenylketonuria, congenital rubella, and Down syndrome. However, a third form has emerged that is being referred to as "acquired or regressive autism" (perhaps the largest subgroup of these children). For purposes of this book, acquired autism is a condition in which the child develops normally for the first twelve to eighteen months of life and then regresses into the increasingly wide spectrum of autistic disorders.

These children challenge the previous belief that 70 to 80 percent of autistic children are mentally challenged. They crawl, sit up, walk, and usually attain normal motor milestones on schedule. Until the age of symptom onset, they are affectionate (which rules out Dr. Kanner's definition) and appear to have above-average intelligence. Children with acquired autism may begin to develop some speech but then, without warning, cease to progress or begin to regress. Suddenly, these children become withdrawn. They vacillate between being quiet and hyperactive. Often self-stimulatory behaviors (e.g., arm flapping, rocking, spinning, or head banging) may develop. Over time, some manifest symptoms that are both similar to and atypical of those of children previously diagnosed as having congenital autism. I propose that many of these children with acquired autism fall into this medical category of NIDS (neuroimmune dysfunction syndromes), and need to be viewed as suffering from an autoimmune medical illness that is potentially treatable.

Understanding, Insight Emerges

To understand how we got here, one has to understand the history. In the early 1970s the human brain was still mainly a black box. There were sophisticated, indirect studies to determine areas of anatomical functions, but the objective data was still essentially nonexistent. We had CAT scans (computed axial tomography) and eventually MRIs (magnetic resonance imaging) capable of illustrating damage, tumors, possible AV (arteriovenous) malformations—essentially what we think of as "structural." There was very little understanding as to the cause of any brain dysfucntion. In fact, in the field of psychiatry, it was generally accepted there was no real objective data, and a whole system of labels and the classification of mental dysfunctions evolved based on symptoms—no one imagined that we'd eventually be able to "look" at how that brain was working or not working.

While specific knowledge was weak (opening up the door to a world classifying many of these disorders, condemning children to a presumed life-term dysfunction, with an absence of objective data), if something was going to go wrong, there were only certain ways that could happen. These children started off with presumed normal brains and normal skulls anatomically; the possible causes of dysfunction are limited.

The possible mechanisms are

1. a structural defect and
2. a congenital/developmental malformation, a chromosome abnormality, an AV or vascular malformation, an injury, a neoplasm/tumor, or a primary metabolic process.

Over many years of study it has been found that none of these possible mechanisms (including any idea of simple genetic or chromosomal defect) is in effect in these children (or adults with these related disorders). The only possibility that remains is that the brain can become dysfunctional by infectious (viral, bacterial, other agents) and immunologic mechanisms. Herpes viruses in particular like to go to the temporal lobe of the brain and are known to cause seizures. Our knowledge of neuroimmune, ultimately complex viral interactions has blossomed because of the appearance of HIV. Short of the indefinable expansion of previous psychiatric-based disorders, one inevitably begins to focus on complex immune and viral mechanisms; that might be a far more reasonable and far more logical explanation than psychiatric/undetectable "developmental" disorders mysteriously present from birth.

The body has different "systems." These include endocrine, immune, hematology, EENT (ear, eye, nose, throat), cardiovascular, pulmonary, GI (gastrointestinal), GU (genital-urinary), muscular-skeletal, and neurological. Within those systems, only certain disease mechanisms can occur. These are metabolic-toxic, genetic/developmental, infectious, immunologic, and tumor-trauma-insult. Looking at these systems, it is obvious by now, while there may be dysfunctions within different body system, the only systems key to the pathophysiology of all this dysfunction/illness are the immunologic and infectious systems. Unless nature and physiology have changed, it's time to focus on reality, science, logic, and a cure.

While in an "ivory tower" medical school—UCLA—I was also thankful upon reflection that I was exposed to the early evolution and understanding of what we called collagen-vascular disorders—things like lupus, scleroderma, and other disorders we now think of as autoimmune diseases. Since we had limited knowledge of our immune system and its complexities, retrospectively it is not a surprise that many markers were not consistently diagnostic or validated as causational. However with ANA and other markers (including abnormal changes in viral titers), we approached patients with an understanding that they could have a potentially serious medical illness.

When I graduated from medical school, the presence of an abnormal immunoglobulin IgM, particularly when elevated, was reason to work up someone for an occult lymphoma or other cancer. Now it is often ignored instead of at least being interpreted as an immune system dysfunction. The cause may not be obvious, but giving these tests as a precaution is a far better, anticipatory, preventative approach than our present system.

When I graduated from medical school, if a young adult developed shingles, (chicken pox reactivation), you would work them up for likelihood of a serious illness, including an occult cancer or leukemia. The reason was that for a young adult to break out in shingles was considered a very serious sign of a stressed immune system. Children, teenagers, and many young adults have this happen now, and are not urgently investigated for a serious illness. Why?

In medical school there was no discussion of entities in adults of chronic fatigue syndrome, fibromyalgia or in children of mixed ADHD, quiet ADHD, or of an epidemic of "autism." As discussed, the appearance of these entities makes sense when looked at together.

It is worth noting that classically autoimmune diseases are more common in women than men, and while "autism" is now in girls and boys, the fact that it is more common in boys than girls may support discussions that boys, before their hormonal changes, may be more susceptible to immune dysfunctions/stress. Perhaps children and adults have been honest when they said they didn't feel good, couldn't think straight, that their brains felt foggy—it turns out that in medical history the mysterious idea of chronic fatigue or CFIDS goes back to at least the 1500s. There have been epidemics throughout history (one documented by the father of English medicine Thomas Siddenhaum in the 1680s) of a mysterious ailment, fatigue, mental dysfunction with a flulike presentation—but unlike today, these presumed outbreaks were reported and then would disappear for long periods of time. Of course with no objective data, no ability to determine the cause of these epidemics, the result was hysteria rather than scientific investigation.

In 1934, Dr. Sandy Gilliam described an outbreak of an unusual fatiguing illness that was then termed "atypical poliomyelitis." Two particular outbreaks that were investigated by Dr. D. A. Henderson at the CDC and Dr. Alexis Shelokov at the NIH led to the term "epidemic neuromyasthenia," which has been the preferred term for outbreaks of fatigue since they reviewed this problem in the *New England Journal of Medicine* back in 1957.

The problem began somewhere in the late 1950s and early 1960s, accelerating dramatically by the 1970s and 1980s. Worldwide outbreaks of this strange phenomenon began to occur, but unlike in the past, they keep recurring, instead of stopping. One of the outbreaks in Japan, in 1984, was termed the "low NK syndrome." Symptoms were a general dullness, with no identifiable bacterial or viral agent evident.

If one applies our emerging understanding of complex immunology and virology, it appears that a medically based epidemic may be occurring—and we have ignored this for at least twenty-six years now.

As far back as an NIH-sponsored research conference in Boston in October 1998, it was acknowledged that some of these "psychosomatic" adults might really have something medically wrong with them. Some of them showed low NK cells, evidence of an immune stress that could lead to chronic viral activation, mitochondrial dysfunction, and unfortunately an increased risk for cancer. At that conference was the recognition that some of these patients were found to have evidence of an "activated" HHV6. Twelve years later, these finding are still being challenged and investigated. Over the years it has remained easier for many in the NIH and our academic institutions to "debate" and challenge viral or immune findings (*they are not the same, they are not consistent on everyone*), rather than focus on explaining and understanding how they might really be playing a key role in the pathogenesis of these disorders. The reasons or explanations for this become harder and harder to understand or remotely justify at a time of crisis like this.

Historically these outbreaks have led to an inquiry and investigation by the NIH's National Institute of Allergy and Infectious Disease and the CDC's Viral Exanthems and Herpesvirus Branch. But unfortunately, CFS/CFIDS was *not* classified as a possible immune or viral disease, and, sadly, high-powered experts concluded these symptoms were psychosomatic. I do not believe we would be missing the medical reality of this misnamed epidemic of "autism" today, if CDC experts, when called in to investigate this outbreak, had been constructive, leading the way on a progressive, logical course to understanding, prevention, and likely treatment. Instead, after first mistakenly dubbing it Epstein-Barr syndrome, due to elevated viral titers, embarrassed, many of the researchers went on personal vendettas, encouraging the press to use the term "yuppie flu," and implying this was not a serious medical illness in these adults (mostly women). It is worth noting that *CFS is no longer considered an infectious disease.* While perhaps not an acute, fast-moving infectious disease like the flu, a cold, measles, or polio, there is no question that we are looking at a slow but insidious immune/viral phenomenon we might have stopped or corrected by now if we had focused resources on understanding, getting answers.

One of the major reasons for the misdirection of the medical system can be traced back to the confusion over the patients presenting during the Lake Tahoe outbreak starting in August/September of 1984. As noted, high-level investigators/researchers disregarded the importance of elevated viral titers. By focusing on psychosomatic causes and ignoring the evidence of viruses and markers for probable immune dysfunction in these adults, we veered off course more than twenty-six years ago.

Back in medical school, we were all taught that evidence for an acute viral infection meant what was called an IgG titer rose, changed fourfold (i.e., 1:20 becomes 1:80 (borderline), 1:40 became 1:160, 1:80 became 1:320, etc.). While not definitive, when symptoms of an illness were present and a viral titer changed fourfold or more, that was considered suggestive, very suspicious evidence for that virus. Even then, without a brain biopsy or a technique that evolved to what we call a positive PCR probe, the titers were suggestive, even convincing, but not definitive proof (the brief appearance of any positive IgM titer was *very* suspicious, often felt to be hard evidence of an active virus—now even that is often ignored as a "false positive"). However, as noted, in 1984 for very complex reasons, when at first these adults and later children appeared with constantly high elevated titers, titers that in medical school we were taught represented presumed evidence of that virus, they were ignored. So instead of what should have been the start of a medical investigation into why these adults had these acutely elevated Epstein-Barr or other viral titers but now on a chronic, long-term basis, mainstream researchers and "medicine" decided (and began to teach) that these titers meant nothing.

Now, instead of twenty-six years devoted to understanding this new disease phenomenon, definitive protocols, and new medications to help, we first discredited adults by calling all their complaints psychosomatic, and now we are somehow selling a completely illogical, unscientific idea that everything in these children is developmental. No.

A recent article from Stanford University illustrates how extreme this has become. A Dr. Montoya and his associates argued that if we were taught that it was significant if viral titers went up fourfold, shouldn't it be significant if *with therapy* the titers went down fourfold? He treated twelve adult, chronically ill CFS/CFIDS patients with elevated herpes-6 (HHV-6) and Epstein-Barr virus (EBV) titers. Each patient had to have four or more of the following neurocognitive symptoms (parents, think of your children): impaired cognitive functioning, slowed processing speed, sleep disturbance, short-term memory deficit, fatigue, and symptoms consistent with depression. After six months with an agent called Valganciclovir (an antiherpes antiviral, but not safe for routine use), nine out of twelve (75 percent) of the patients experienced near resolution of their symptoms, resumed daily home and/or work functions—something they had been unable to do for years.

In a world that denies meaning to these titers in adults and children, the researchers showed a significant drop in both their EBV VCA IgG titers (1:2560 > 1:640) and their HHV-6 IgG titers (1:1280 > 1:320).

Key researchers I've been involved with, who are openly pleased with "the Dr. Montoya article" acknowledged they could never have received funding or approval in the current research atmosphere. Only because he was so powerful, so "big," was he able to do it. After twenty-six years of this, isn't it time the prevailing attitudes changed?

3

○ ○ ○ ◎ ◉ ◎ ○ ○

CHANGING LETTERS:
ADD? ADHD? MIXED ADHD?
QUIET ADD?

I N THE EARLY TO MID 1980s, the varying labels of ADHD (ADD with hyperactivity, ADD without hyperactivity, ADHD, etc.) were being applied to describe the newly dysfunctional children appearing in my practice and around the country. With no imaging and no application of new tools to understand the brain, the radical differences with the new ADHD (now the majority in pediatrics) have not been understood—leading to likely medication errors in these children. Making judgments, even educated ones, based on symptomatology, without closer evaluation of real function in the brain, in my opinion, should not be allowed in the twenty-first century. We now have the tools. We have a responsibility to use them. From NeuroSPECT work (see later discussion in this book and article references), the old-fashioned hyper-ADHD child (bright, alert, with increased blood flow to the frontal lobes and normal temporal lobes and rest of brain) is quite different from the new mixed or quiet ADHDs (where each has components of temporal lobe hypoperfusion, and usually has components of "spaciness," "zoniness," cognitive dysfunctions, anxiety, oppositional behaviors, or depression).

With this insight, the obvious idea is that this is not the same as whatever was happening with the possible 5–10 percent of children, usually boys, who were considered the old-fashioned hyper-ADD child. As noted, that child was bright, intelligent, and alert—if you could get them in their seats. Significantly, there was no discussion in medical school of these children having cognitive or executive dysfunction. Subsequently, on NeuroSPECT scans, they had hyperperfusion in their frontal lobes and a generally healthy rest of the brain. When the mixed, quiet, and multiple other variants of ADHD began to appear, it was immediately obvious—since most of them had components of temporal lobe dysfunction, temporal lobe hypoperfusion—something else must be going on.

Against this background of an autism epidemic, attention deficits now represents not only the most common developmental problem in school-age children but has also changed dramatically. Where it was once thought that ADD affected school-age children, who were expected to outgrow their "ADD" issues by puberty, it is now recognized that between 50 to 70 percent of children with attention deficits diagnosed between six and twelve years of age continue to manifest troublesome symptoms throughout adolescence and beyond. With the term ADHD now routinely applied to adults and children, and with multiple variants discussed, perhaps it is time to recognize that this has nothing to do with the original work about ADD/ADHD. An increasing number of ADHD children are now being diagnosed with Tourette's syndrome. Tourette is now viewed as "immune" related. I not only believe that none of this is coincidental but also that the only way to understand it is the overwhelming fact we have an unrecognized medical epidemic. This is not compatible with the idea of suddenly better awareness, or as noted, an "epidemic" of previous developmental or psychological categories of dysfunction.

Supporting the conclusion that this is a new medical epidemic are observations by researchers over the last three decades that continue to emphasize the contribution of weaknesses in higher-order cognitive functions (i.e., thinking and reasoning processes) to the school failure of many learning-disabled children. Children have appeared in large numbers with deficits in "metacognitive" skills (i.e., being able to access acquired knowledge when needed, knowing how to apply learned skills). These children are unable to focus their attention on the salient features of tasks. They cannot effectively devise strategies to get them done. These children are often described as "passive" learners. It was immediately obvious that when I was taught that an ADD child (referred to as hyper-ADD) was inherently very intelligent, very bright, "they just could not be kept in their seats," it was clearly a different era, and those children presented with different symptoms than they have now. Children now present with cognitive issues, and these children are appearing in larger and larger numbers. These symptoms, these ADHD variants that were not even recognized in the 1970s, are now the vast majority. We are also, to our great detriment as a society, continuing to focus on all the "other" reasons why schools are failing, grades are falling, IQs are *dropping*, without any recognition that these children are having an outright "cognitive dysfunction" from a disease. How long do we fail, and how long do we allow these children to fail, before we say enough is enough?

With the rapidly enlarging group of children that do not fit "classic" autistic profiles, the number of ADHD variants, and other multiple labels being used to categorize, define our children, it is time to step back, and return these children to the medical world. With the increased recognition and understanding of immune-dysregulatory phenomenon, it is time to realize these issues in children are not secondary to some strange, previously misunderstand developmental or psychological issues, but we have a real medical epiphenomenon. Whether this epiphenomenon is caused by a retrovirus, a regular virus, a genetic disposition (very probable), environmental changes (very probable), ozone layer issues, or multiple other factors insinuated or looked at over the years impacting our immune systems, once in effect we have a process being controlled by the body's own "innate" neuroimmune system (supported by multiple peer-reviewed articles), and it's time we understood that and dealt with that appropriately and effectively as medical physicians.

Additional support for the immune system linkage, not as a secondary factor but as a true primary pathophysiologic explanation for this disease/disorder, is the recognition that within this group of patients a common denominator is a large number of allergies or intolerances. Around 25 percent of healthy children now have chronic illnesses including allergies, migraines, diabetes, and more, while it has been also recognized that many children with complex medical disorders show allergies and immune issues. Commonly, within the family histories one often finds eczema, migraines (especially in mothers), hay fever, asthma, and/or some other "autoimmune" disease such as thyroiditis, lupus, or rheumatoid arthritis. As I point out to parents frequently, this supports the primary pathophysiology of the immune system, immune-related issues, not something being developmental or genetic. What one does not see within these families is a routine history of true genetic or developmental disorders.

How is it that nobody has recognized or linked the lowering of IQ over the last twenty years per ERIC (Educational Resource Information Center) databases to the likelihood of a medical, cognitive, and physical epidemic?

As noted elsewhere, the key is the recognition that these new type of children with ADHD, Tourette's syndrome, and other variants of LD (learning disorders) really had a common denominator of temporal lobe hypoperfusion, linked, one could argue, by the new idea we were proposing called NIDS.

Going beyond just the study of symptoms and intelligent but subjective ideas and approximations, this gave a logical, objective insight to understand these disorders and, most important, look at real treatment goals for these children. (Again, the fact that our medical system is still pursuing subjective treatment and medications for these children should be intolerable to all parents of children afflicted with these disorders.)

While I was generally opposed to the use of stimulant medications for something we called hyper ADD, and though I was never comfortable with not understanding how they worked, it turns out in some situations they might have helped that child with "classic" hyper ADD. That said, the chances of helping the new "mixed" or quiet type of ADD via these methods are not only extremely low, in theory they may be causing long-term harm. Based on NeuroSPECT, as noted, the original class ADD child had too *much* function, with increased blood flow in their frontal lobes. While I remain generally opposed to their use, one could argue that stimulant medications, with their now recognized vasoconstrictive action (just like cocaine and amphetamines), had a limited place in the treatment of those type of children. One was potentially decreasing blood flow to those hot frontal lobes with, one hopes, minimal negative effects to the key temporal lobes. The problem is that even today, it is difficult to conceive of long-term "cocaine use" (i.e., the effects of ritalin or amphetamine-based medications today) ever being healthy for the brain. In fact, while I was in medical school these "upper" stimulant medications that calmed hyperactive children down were not recommended with teenagers or adults. We were warned not to use them in teenagers or adults. How is it that they are routinely being used in adolescents and adults today? Instead of using stimulant medications as prescription uppers for a seemingly tired brain, perhaps it's time we asked why these patients are tired and why they have trouble staying focused. If we did, maybe we would understand that we are looking at a medically based disorder, not the developmental disorder of decades ago. Like autism, and now autism spectrum disorder, we have expanded almost exponentially the labels (based on combinations of symptoms) rather than look at a true medical, physiologically based disorder or problem.

The problem was soon quite obvious. Approaching the expanding categories of ADHD in a knee-jerk manner, we are using stimulant medications (although some experts are finally beginning to change) for these new kinds of ADDs, just like the hyper-ADDs. In these children, one could first argue theoretically, using a vasoconstrictor (which causes a narrowing of the arteries), like a stimulant medication, particularly without an SSRI or other support for the temporal lobes, could very likely result in a net ongoing education dysfunction, and even a lowering of IQ potential, by further slowing down or delaying already-decreased temporal lobe functions.

Sadly, these concerns are probably no longer idle or just theoretical, because if you look at the statistics around this country, there is now a recognized lowering of the IQ potential of children across many grade levels. How many adolescents (perhaps at that age still more boys than girls) are not really healthy, not energetic or sharp enough to really push themselves to excel? How many are part of our growing rate of high school dropouts? If they make it to college, how many of these young adults are unable to function in a college environment, after going through high school on stimulant medications, perhaps seeming to do okay, but likely missing many key cognitive tools they were supposed to have developed further or better? The good and the bad here is that with many years of insight and good scientific studies, we now know the brain is more pliable than we imagined—able to develop years beyond old ideas, old time lines. It is just as correct to say that we are not born with a five- or ten-year-old brain. We have known for years that the brain is like a muscle. As we mature, as we use it, we develop new tracks, we refine connections to become more efficient, faster, etc. Beyond just not functioning right, it has become apparent that we are missing key maturation and development points when an area is shut down, not functioning correctly. So only by directing appropriate therapies can we realistically hope to allow these areas to reopen, regain potential ability, and function in a healthier manner. Only then, for so many of these interconnected cognitive disorders, do you have any real expectation, potential chance, or possible true goal of restoring function and higher developmental abilities. Everything happening makes sense if we look at this as an illness and apply hard science.

4

A HISTORY OF
MEDICAL RESEARCH

A REVIEW OF THE EXISTING MEDICAL LITERATURE relative to autism research reveals evidence of an emerging medical disease *process* in these children. For instance, research indicates that autism can follow infectious disorders affecting the central nervous system including encephalitis.[1, 2, 3, 4] Multiple studies have focused on various anatomic locations of suspected dysfunction.[5, 6, 7, 8] It is important to note that emphasis is often put on the medial temporal lobe. Pertinent to this new "model" of dysfunction are the multiple published reports of autistic symptoms developing in association with encephalitis in children.[9] Most of these reports cite injury to the temporal lobes as part of their findings. This is consistent with the areas of decreased function identified on NeuroSPECT scans initially working with a Dr. Ismael Mena and a Dr. Bruce Miller at HGH-UCLA, and now continuing with Dr. Mena (long distance from Chile, no less) and a Dr. Michael Uszler, based in Santa Monica. Interestingly, along the way we've had a few doctors involved who, with some exposure to our research seemed to go from open skeptics to scientists recognizing the existence of a problem worth further research and investigation. It all comes back to restrictions of our system; we can't open up new answers, get to understanding, if we are not willing to use or accept new tools, offering potentially new, objective information about the "black box" we have called the brain. Restricting most studies, particularly the very large NIH-sponsored study looking at a large number of children and their families, to MRIs, or CAT scans, or other markers and tests I was taught to use thirty years ago, is saying that while we have a major crisis, and while we are going to commit major resources to it, we are going to make sure we cannot get any really new information or new data that might undermine old ideas. This approach is frightening and should be of great concern to others out there looking for help and potential new answers.

New research techniques are increasing the rates at which herpes simplex virus (HSV) sequences are being identified in temporal lobe tissues[10, 11,] (i.e., locales likely to be substrates for various aspects of autism). In 1975, an article was published in *Cortex*[12] describing a syndrome similar to autism in adult psychiatry. The condition involves the loss of emotional significance of objects, the inability to adapt in social settings, the loss of recognition of the significance of persons, and the absence of sustained purposeful activity *after temporal lobe damage.*

The literature also comments on the cognitive and behavioral deficits caused by temporal lobe damage in herpes encephalitis. There are many reports, particularly in the British literature,[13] suggesting a connection to coxsackie/enteroviruses, while in the United States it has been suggested that many cases may be linked to the herpes family of viruses (i.e., EBV, HHV6, HHV7, CMV, etc.).[14, 15, 16, 17, 18] Neither theory has been conclusively proven, nor has the evidence for a contagious disorder been conclusive (although some have inferred it based upon incidents related to epidemic outbreaks[19, 20]). However, HSV in humans has long been known to prefer temporal lobe and limbic sites. One theory focuses on the olfactory nerves as a possible route for infection, but oral cavities may also provide entry. In 1996, O'Meara et al. postulated the following: "Inoculation of murine tooth pulp with HSV selectively infected the mandibular division of the trigeminal nerve and caused encephalitis predominantly affecting the temporal cortex and limbic system, a pattern of disease similar to human HSE [herpes simplex encephalitis]".[21]

While other studies have also implicated the temporal lobes in the pathogenesis of autism,[22, 23] a direct association between temporal lobe pathology and autism has not yet been proven conclusively. In fact, research has found a variety of lesions in the "autistic" brain, particularly in the cerebellum.[24] These variable findings may be due to the heterogeneity (differences) in the possible etiologies or time/duration effects within this syndrome.

Although herpes viruses have a predilection for the temporal lobes,[25] the course of autism does not suggest an acute infection with traditional herpes viruses.[26] However, delayed temporal lobe development early in life may produce different symptoms from those arising from deterioration or destruction of previously normal lobes.

In summary, although not conclusive, past research further strengthens the linkage of the temporal lobe and "autistic" symptoms. Boucher and Warrington noted similarities between behavioral deficits reported in animals with hippocampal lesions and autistic behavior.[27] Medial temporal lobe damage on pneumoencephalograms was reported in a subset of autistic children.[28] Damasio and Mauer proposed that "the syndrome results from dysfunction in a system of bilateral neural structures that includes the ring of mesolimbic cortex located in the mesial frontal and temporal lobes, the neostriatum, and the anterior and medial nuclear groups of the thalamus." At least two other studies have also implicated the temporal lobes in the pathogenesis of autism.[29, 30]

5

THE EVIDENCE

WITH NEW AND MORE PRECISE TOOLS and technology available to us now, the medical anatomy of "autism" is gaining definition after years of conflicting findings. Currently, EEG abnormalities,[1] immune markers, and NeuroSPECT findings support the concept of a medical disease process occurring in these children's brains. For example, it is generally recognized that an EEG finding of "slow" waves or "abnormal" brain wave activity is often consistent with the idea of an underlying and unknown encephalopathy/encephalitis.

In addition, ongoing work with the NeuroSPECT strengthens the connection of blood flow abnormalities and neurodysfunctional states, particularly in situations in which patients appear to have immune and/or possible viral etiologies. NeuroSPECT scans capture blood flow through specific areas of the brain. Blood flow correlates with function/activity.[2, 3] As noted, NeuroSPECT scans on children with autism have shown a decrease in blood flow in the temporal and occipital areas, which is consistent with past reports of temporal lobe dysfunction in such children. Neurological models of the brain correlate right temporal lobe areas with social skills and left temporal lobe areas with speech and auditory processing, all of which are compromised in autistic children. It should also be noted that there is no good explanation for our finding of increased blood flow in the frontal lobes of a group of these children, which is more consistent with ADD and hyperactivity. Further research is required relative to this finding.

When monitoring the emerging body of evidence related to the immune system and its interactive messengers, interleukins and cytokines, it appears that a dysregulated immune system state—whether triggered by a virus, genetic disposition, or intrauterine, prenatal, or neonatal stress or trauma—may account for the cognitive processing and other deficits seen in some children with autism. This concept is supported by the lack of consistent neurological/anatomical abnormalities and metabolic abnormalities in these children. We now know that neuropolypeptides called cytokines can and do restrict brain blood flow under certain conditions. In these children, we may be looking at an immune system continually sending out signals to restrict brain blood flow. Whether this continues as an autoimmune reaction (whereby the immune system continues this pathway with no active reason to do so) or is due to the presence of a retroviral or other viral process is open to further research. However, the concept of an immune-related disease process in a large number of these children appears unquestionable at this point in time.

Many autistic children have major allergies or intolerances to many chemicals and foods. While occasionally these reactions may turn into urticaria or asthma, the effect in the majority of these children is the worsening of autistic-like behavior. Family history often reveals eczema, migraines (especially in mothers), hay fever, asthma, and histories of other disorders, which are often immune-mediated. These external symptoms may well prove to be signs of a hyper-reactive/stressed/dysfunctional immune system underlying the biochemistry of these children. Many anecdotal reports of successful therapies for autistic children (e.g., gammaglobulin, allergy-free diets) can most likely be explained through the concept of regulating a dysfunctional immune system and/or altering metabolic sensitivities and dysfunction.

Examples of autism's probable connection to immune dysfunctional states are seen in the following:

Extensive clinical work over the last four to five years further supports the hypothesis that we are facing an immune-mediated disease state affecting the central nervous system (CNS) in these children. The literature is replete with articles connecting immune system abnormalities to autism, ADD, ADHD, CFS, and CFIDS. Here are several main examples:

1. Multiple researchers have found evidence that autoimmunity is a possible mechanism to explain autistic symptoms.[4, 5, 6, 7, 8]

2. An increased incidence of two or more miscarriages and infertility[9,] as well as preeclampsia[10] and bleeding during pregnancy[11] has been shown to occur in mothers of autistic children. There are also multiple studies in the obstetrical literature connecting these events to immune autoantibody production.

3. Studies have been done comparing the maternal antibodies of mothers with their autistic children,[12] suggesting an association of abnormal maternal immunity with autism. Antibodies reactive with lymphocytes of fathers of autistic children have also been found.

Multiple researchers have shown an interaction of maternal antibodies with trophoblast or embryonic tissue antigens, and a cross-reaction with antigens found on lymphocytes.[13, 14, 15, 16]

Researchers have also shown a significant depression of CD4+ T helper cells and their suppresser-inducer subset[17, 18] with an increased frequency of the null allele at the complement C4B locus[19] in children with autism. As similar changes have been known to occur in other autoimmune diseases,[20, 21] these researchers have postulated that immune activation of a T cell subpopulation may be important in the etiology of the disorder in some children with autism. Note: Many of the autistic children evaluated in studies and within my practice have shown very high CD4 and CD8 counts, low natural killer (NK) cells, or other "markers" consistent with immune dysfunction/dysregulation.

Abnormalities of cell adhesion molecules (NCAM)[22] have been reported.

Antibodies to neurofilament axonal proteins (NFAP) have been noted in autistic children[23] and have been reported in neurotropic "slow virus" diseases (kuru and Creutzfeldt-Jakob disease) in adults.[24] Other studies[25, 26] have suggested an association of an infectious agent (slow virus) in the etiology of these diseases. This is considered indirect evidence that some cases of autism may also be associated with the concept of a slow virus.

Anti–central nervous system serum immunoglobin reactivity has been reported that was specifically directed against the cerebellum.[27]

A small percentage of autistic children with demonstrable immunologic abnormalities have normalized their autistic symptoms with intravenous immunoglobulin treatment.[28, 29] This result shows that immune abnormalities can cause autism in a subset of children and that acquired autism can be effectively treated.

Singh et al. hypothesized that autoimmunity secondary to a virus infection may best explain autism in some children.[30] Congenital rubella virus[31] and congenital cytomegalovirus[32] have been indirectly involved as causative factors in autism.

Given this support and much more from the medical research literature, the concept of immune dysregulation as a medical disease process in childhood neurocognitive dysfunction is an emerging reality. This concept could easily account for a significant portion of the increase of neurocognitive diagnoses over the last twenty to thirty years. Whether the etiology of this dysfunction is related to environmental factors (e.g., ozone layer depletion, local toxins, etc.), new retroviruses, or stealth, spongiform or other viruses (or altered viral responses), we now have a medical hypothesis that can facilitate the definition of clinical subgroups and lead to the treatment of these patients without first determining the exact/specific origin or etiology.

If an infectious etiology indeed exists, it may be as ordinary as the common cold or so rare that we have not yet developed the tools to identify or study it. Whether an ongoing agent is present, or the body simply remains in a dysfunctional state, it seems likely we are confronted with a phenomenon/illness that has multiple etiologies, multiple origins, and various clinical manifestations. At this point, they appear linked by an immune dysfunction or possible viral-mediated state. Genetic predisposition to this syndrome may have a great deal to do with why certain individuals suffer with these symptoms. However, we must begin to consider these apparently heterogeneous expressions as linked and potentially treatable through the common pathway of an immune dysfunctional/CNS dysregulated state. For example, in a study[33] on chronic fatigue syndrome (CFS), Dr. Mena and I reported a significant diminution of blood flow in both the temporal and, to a lesser degree, the parietal lobes in children suffering from CFS and chronic fatigue immune dysfunction syndrome (CFIDS). These findings are similar to those previously noted in children with acquired autism.

The ASD medical disease hypothesis began to take form in the 1980s when multiple researchers found evidence that autoimmunity was a possible mechanism to explain autistic symptoms.[37,38,39,40,41] Since these initial observations, the body of evidence has grown dramatically—witness this statement from Johns Hopkins Department of Neurology website (December 2009):

> Current evidence suggests that neurobiological abnormalities in autism are associated with changes in cytoarchitectural and neuronal organization that may be determined by genetic, environmental, immunological, and toxic factors. Since neuroglia has central roles during brain development, cortical organization, neuronal function and immune responses, we hypothesize that neuroglia may contribute to the pathogenesis of autism in several ways:
>
> Neuroglia may be dysfunctional during the process of neuronal organization and plasticity of cortical and subcortical structures, a change that may contribute to the neuropathological abnormalities observed in autism.
>
> Neuroglia may react to extrinsic factors, such as systemic immune responses, toxins, or infections, and produce disturbances in the CNS microenvironment that facilitate the development of immune-mediated reactions.
>
> Abnormal neuroglial activation may be present in autistic patients due to genetic susceptibility to inflammation, a change that can lead to abnormalities in neuronal-neuroglial interactions.
>
> Neuroglial activation can trigger the development of cellular or humoral immune responses that lead to neuronal/neuroglial dysfunction.

1. *Systemic immune responses may trigger abnormal pathogenic reactions in neuroglia.*

Our experimental approaches include study of brain tissues obtained from patients with autism, determination of the profile of cytokines and chemokines and characterization of immune-mediated reactions in cortical and subcortical regions of autistic brains. Further understanding of the role of neuroglia and immune reactions in the neurobiology of autism may contribute to the design of therapeutic interventions that minimize the neurological and behavioral abnormalities that occur in this disease.

The cornerstone research was published in two journals ("Brain Inflammation Is a Sign of Autism," *Annals of Neurology*, 15 November 2004; 01:18 and "Immunity, Neuroglia and Neuroinflammation in Autism," *Internet Review of Psychiatry*, December 2005; 17[6]: 485–495). The study demonstrated the presence of neuroglial and innate neuroimmune system activation in brain tissue and cerebrospinal fluid of patients with autism, findings that support the view that neuroimmune abnormalities occur in the brains of autistic patients and may contribute to the diversity of the autistic phenotypes.

Here are multiple other studies that almost indisputably point to NIDS (or an immune-mediated encephalopathy) as playing a role in children and adults now labeled ASD:

Science reported in October 2009 that a relatively new retrovirus, XMRV, was identified in a higher-than-normal proportion of CFS patients, and also reported similar findings for people with autism, atypical multiple sclerosis, and fibromyalgia ("Detection of an Infectious Retrovirus, XMRV, in Blood Cells of Patients with Chronic Fatigue Syndrome," *Science* Magazine New York, New York, Published Online, October 8, 2009).

In February 2009, the *Journal of Neuroimmunology* published a study concluding that ASD patients displayed an increased innate and adaptive immune response through the Th1 pathway, suggesting that localized brain inflammation and autoimmune disorder may be involved in the pathogenesis of ASD ("Elevated Immune Response in the Brain of Autistic Patients," *Journal of Neuroimmunology.* 2009 Feb 15: 207 [1–2]: 111–6 Epub 2009 Jan).

These 2007 studies measured the presence of autoantibodies (directed against neural antigens) in ASD patients and explored the possible role of autoimmunity in the pathogenesis of ASD ("Brain-Specific Autoantibodies in the Plasma of Subjects with Autistic Spectrum Disorder," *Annals of the New York Academy of Science,* 2007 Jun; 1107:92–103 and "Autoantibodies in Autism Spectrum Disorders," *Annals of the New York Academy of Science,* 2007 Jun: 1107:79–91).

- During embryogenesis, unregulated VIP may have major and permanent consequences on the formation of the brain and may be a participating factor in disorders of neurodevelopment. VIP has been linked to autism, Down syndrome, and fetal alcohol syndrome ("Vasoactive Intestinal Peptide in Neurodevelopmental Disorders: Therapeutic Potential," Current Pharmaceutical Design. 2007 13[11]: 1079–89).
- This research indicates that there is potential that aberrant immune activity during vulnerable and critical periods of neurodevelopment could participate in the generation of neurological dysfunction characteristic of ASD ("The Immune Response in Autism: A New Frontier for Autism Research," *Journal of Leukocyte Biology.* 2006 80[1]: 1–15. Epub May 12 2006).
- In this 2006 review, immune abnormalities are also commonly observed in this disorder. Given 5-HT's role as an immunomodulator, possible connections between 5-HT and immune abnormalities in autism are explored ("Hyperserotoninemia and Altered Immunity in Autism," *Journal of Autism and Developmental Disorders.* 2006 July 36[5]: 697–704).
- The presence of both BDNF AAs and elevated BDNF levels in some children with autism and childhood disintegrative disorder suggests a previously unrecognized interaction between the

immune system and BDNF ("Brain-Derived Neurotrophic Factor and Autoantibodies to Neural Antigens in Sera of Children with Autism Spectrum Disorders, Landau-Kleffner Syndrome, and Epilepsy," Biology Psychiatry. 2006 Feb 15; 59(4): 354–63. Epub September 21 2005).

- Two main immune dysfunctions in autism are immune regulation involving proinflammatory cytokines (immunomodulating agents) and autoimmunity. Studies showing elevated brain specific antibodies in autism support an autoimmune mechanism. Viruses may initiate the process but the subsequent activation of cytokines is the damaging factor associated with autism.[34]

Among the main immune abnormalities reported:

Changes in T cells (and T cell function)
CD4/CD8—increased/decreased
Low (and elevated) NK cells
B cells—increased/decreased
Increased DR+ T cells
Increased interleukin-2 receptors
Decreased mitogen response
Altered delayed hypersensitivity
Antibodies to serotonin receptors
Antibodies to neuro elements

Based on the evidence presented herein, I believe that developing a focus on the interrelationship of autism, ADD, ADHD, CFS, CFIDS, and other immune-modulated conditions is a key to helping groups of these children in ways never before possible. If we can address the physiologic part of the dysfunction in these children (irrespective of its specific etiology), educational therapy, counseling, study techniques, and most/all other current therapies have a far greater probability of success. In addition, research focused on developing and initiating new therapies for "autism" is likely to be useful in treating these other interrelated childhood disorders.

Seizures—Relationship to Viruses, Immune Attacks on Brain

Years ago in medical school, we were taught that a certain number of pediatric patients were going to have febrile seizures. They were otherwise presumed to be healthy, and they would progress to develop correctly, and essentially outgrow their tendency to "febrile seizures." Most seizures, even in later childhood, were considered idiopathic (from an unknown cause).

In the last few years, besides all the children now diagnosed as having "autism with seizures," I began to meet parents of children presenting with one hundred or more seizures a month, sometimes one hundred a week. As any doctor will tell you—this many childhood seizures would ordinarily be diagnosed as a neurological (not psychiatric) disorder called epilepsy. Yet, to my surprise and dismay, these parents were distraught, as lost as parents of "autistic" children, for they were being told by the top pediatric neurologists in the country that their children's seizures were idiopathic.

I knew there was an enlarging body of good, peer-reviewed evidence that a new family of higher-order herpes viruses, HHV-6, HHV-7, HHV-8 and more, were unlike the herpes simplex viruses so many of us were taught about in medical school. These viruses wanted to go to the brain, but unlike previous models, previous teaching, they smoldered at a low grade (below the radar—stealthily). Since I had never been told a virus living on my brain was good for me, besides the explanation for the neurodysfunction evolving in adults and then children, the idea of viruses was a perfect explanation for increased seizures. As noted below, the addition of the immune system itself attacking the brain completed a picture, compatible with medical school teaching, of what we were told were "irritable foci." When they fire off inappropriately the brain could then fire off inappropriately at large, creating a seizure!

In preparing to give a talk to these parents I was floored, then dismayed, that in peer-reviewed medical journals talking about seizures, the literature was not only full of neuroimmune, chemokines, cytokines, but by the literature at least 25 to perhaps as many as 40 percent of these children had evidence for herpes viruses in their brain, particularly the temporal lobes. The concept of the temporal lobes, herpes viruses, and seizure foci has been strengthened over the years by repeatedly confirmed findings on autopsies in children and adults. As noted above, we know HHV-6 and related viruses go to the brain. A very disturbing finding in the literature was the fact that latent (30 percent) and active (12 percent) forms of HHV-6 were found in supposedly "normal" pediatric brains on autopsy. The article stongly supported the idea that "the glial tropism and anatomical location of HHV-6 may have important implications into the pathogenesis of disease." How can we tell so many parents their children's seizures are idiopathic and accept missing so many likely reasons and pathogens? Again, by a system not willing to put any "marker" value on elevated titers, with the fallacies of PCR probes (which will be positive sometimes, but not consistently), short of brain biopsies, how do we verify, prove what should be clinically obvious to many by now?

In using NeuroSPECT for many years now, it has become obvious that "scattered" areas of dysfunction, vasculitis with either increased or decreassd flow, was occurring in areas that could not be correlated to existing tracks or pathways in the brain. The findings over many years now are only consistent with the idea of a virus scattered living in/irritating the brain, and/or the immune system attacking those or other scattered areas of the brain.

Case note: A ten-year-old old girl, presenting with epilepsy and autism, had NK cells of 2.8 percent, a sedimentation rate of one. With those findings alone, irrespective of other parts of her history, the likelihood she was in a neuroimmune state, had a stressed immune system, and an overwhelming probability of viral activation was clinically a sure thing. Whatever the original reason, or insult, this said there was something medically going on that I was likely familiar with, and I could likely try to help this patient. I am pleased to say, over a year later, with The Goldberg Approach (see chapter 7) seizures are almost nonexistent, negative medications are lower or removed, and she is beginning to blossom educationally and physically, as she never could before.

Reviewing the seizure literature, it turned out there were many articles supporting the potential role for herpes-related viruses, including a number on the likely role of HHV-6b in epilepsy, limbic encephalitis, myocarditis, encephalitis, febrile seizures, and MS.

Clinical Note: As a general pediatrician, before subspecializing, I had become aware that newly identified HHV-6, the common cause of roseola in children, was possibly connected to febrile seizures.

Many articles supported these ideas, these connections, but it was becoming obvious, even for university-based pediatric neurologists, this was a direction they were not pursuing. It is worth noting that often the articles refer to the lack of conventional inflammatory changes, which is to me completely supportive of the idea of neuroimmunity being presented in this book.

With the literature validating that many febrile seizures are occurring without the previous concept of a rapid rise in temperature, understanding that many of these are not benign anymore, that many are forerunners to true epilepsy, potentially lifelong seizure disorders, mean therapy and prevention need to come to the forefront, not just watchful waiting; these "idiopathic" seizures are perhaps no longer really benign.

Along with the multiple articles or various roles of the immune system and chemokine and cytokine abnormalities related to seizures came a very interesting finding. In the "epilepsy and seizure" literature articles showed a direct linkage of the concept of peripheral inflammation mediating or leading to altered CNS excitability.[35] It was shown that in a mouse or rat given a chemical causing GI inflammation, an increased susceptibility to seizures "strongly correlated with the severity and progression of intestinal inflammation." If we're not looking at proper dietary controls, if we're giving impure supplements or agents that may be allergenic to a child, how much harm will be done? Worse, does the recognition of GI inflammation leading to brain inflammation confirm another likely cause, besides just viral, for the disproportionately large increase in seizures in "autistic" children?

This area needs a full pediatric investigation immediately. Inadvertently, many parents may be being asked to do things that are not only not helping, but may be contributing to increased long-term dysfunction and morbidity. While frustrated (to say the least) by the failure of current researchers to recognize that autism in the past had essentially *no* association with seizures; now when 35–40 percent of children with "autism" are prone to seizures, how much longer is it going to take to realize there is no relationship between what is happening now, and whatever we thought this was in the past?

Within the seizure literature, they are already looking at creative ways to reduce inflammation and block or prevent the attacks on the brain, I continue to believe that within this medical specialty, stepping back, looking at the bigger picture of that child and his or her general health, immunity, and brain could be a big step forward.

From a disorder being called "autism" in the 1940s and 1950s with no connection of note to seizures in those children presenting then, to the routine statement that 35–40 percent of these children today may develop seizures, is one very large additional finding that should clearly demonstrate this is not Dr. Kanner's autism.

Pituitary—Hypothalamic Growth

Over the years, consistent with the medical world documenting a significant increase in thyroid disorders in adults and children, growth disorders in children, and other pituitary/endocrine disorders in general, came the recognition and understanding that the findings on NeuroSPECT, the neuroimmune-mediated shutdown of blood flow and function going on in the temporal lobes of the brain could begin to explain some of the enlarging endocrine dysfunction that was occuring. In particular, this could explain the increasing number of cases pediatric endocrinologists were seeing and calling "atypical." More than a decade ago, I had some very interesting discussion with top pediatric endocrinologists regarding mutual patients that were having "baffling" growth issues. Pituitary markings/findings might make sense if they thought of the general "pituitary-hypothalamic" system as not broken, but dysfunctional—thankfully this was logical to them.

> To a pediatrician, always aware of growth and development in a child, aware of expected markers or ways to detect dysfunction, it became obvious that not only were there real issues for children from GH (growth hormone) dysfunction, but as I would frequently advice a parent whose child was being evaluated but who we knew had NIDS, neuroimmune issues, that just a "static" test of growth hormone function would often be normal, when a stressed or dynamic one would be abnormal. This becomes logical in terms of a system that is not broken, but is dysfunctional.

Over the years the idea of autoimmune, dysfunctional, but not broken was illustrated by the classical teaching of thyroiditis and its ability to result in increased and/or decreased function, depending upon the disease process, and activity levels. That was not the teaching for much of what we called pituitary disorders, but now the neuroimmune connection may begin to explain a lot of what has certainly been perplexing to pediatric patients and their endocrinologists.

6

NEUROSPECT: A NEW TOOL

A NEW DIAGNOSTIC TOOL FOR UNDERSTANDING THE brain has emerged over the past two decades called NeuroSPECT. SPECT stands for *s*ingle *p*hoton *e*mission *c*omputed *t*omography. It is a sophisticated nuclear medicine study that looks directly at the cerebral blood flow in the brain and indirectly at brain activity.

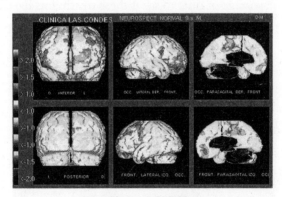
A normal NeuroSPECT scan

How Does It Work?

A radioactive isotope is injected into a patient's vein and then runs through the bloodstream and is taken up by receptors in the brain. A state-of-the-art camera, designed to detect where the compound has gone in the brain, captures these images and in conjunction with a computer creates maps blood flow, which correlates directly to brain activity. In other words, we can now witness changes in increased and decreased function in different areas of the brain, including deep inside the brain. While now PET scans can give ideas of function also, to this day, NeuroSPECT is considered to be consistently more objective and reproducible overall (especially with new computerized software).

What Does This Mean?

Everyone by now is familiar with CAT scans and MRI scans. These scans offer images of a static brain and its anatomy; they are great for seeing growths and injury but not useful for seeing activity (blood flow) in a working brain—in other words, how a brain functions. By comparing SPECT images of healthy brains with dysfunctional brains, we can accurately identify the disease processes taking place in immune-stressed brains. These SPECT scans illuminate such neuroimmune system dysfunctions as attention deficit disorder (ADD), autism, and chronic fatigue syndrome. We can finally see what is going wrong, which contributes hugely to both our understanding and the development of treatment plans that can treat these problems. What's more, we can rescan after some appropriate passage of time to see if these treatments have been effective, thus providing physical validation of the efficacy of various treatments!

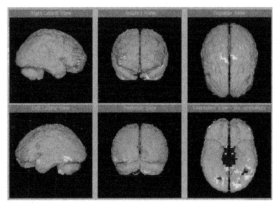

A child doing very well, with "The Goldberg Approach™" (still some frontal hyperness)

Impact

This is a first in human history. The brain has been a black box sitting on top of our necks, in charge of everything and a complete mystery, because we couldn't see into it. We have been making inroads over the last few years with such tools as CAT scans and PET scans and MRIs . But this is the first time we can physically correlate brain activity with behavior. Now we can *see* the part(s) of the brain that are dysfunctional, and so if you have ADD-HD, if your child has autism, if your partner is suffering with chronic fatigue syndrome, we can see how that disease manifests in the brain. While debates continue between proponents of PET and proponents of NeuroSPECT, for now, SPECT continues to have an edge in reproducibility and objectivity for these types of disorders.

With Dr. Ismael Mena and Dr. Bruce Miller, I had a very unique opportunity, not usually possible outside a private practice. When I first began looking at these disorders, it was becoming obvious that the common link with the brain was the immune system. As a clinician, I will state strongly that nothing else could make sense and tie the various presentations together except a common denominator, the brain-immune system. This concept was firmly supported when at the first DAN organizational meeting in Dallas, in 1995, I watched Dr. Sudhir Gupta, a heavily certified adult immunologist, go up to the board and cross out multiple arrows referring to the body and presumed pathways, leaving only: *brain—immune system.*

When I met Dr. Mena and became aware of his advanced work with NeuroSPECT imaging, it was the end of any further debate. The NeuroSPECT objectively showed blood flow in the brain, which translates accurately to function. As a private physician, I was able to send children and some adults for scans, procedures approved even by Blue Cross-Blue Shield insurance plans at the time, which would have been considered "experimental" and probably never authorized were I working in a university position. And I will never forget when I met Dr. Bruce Miller, considered a world leader, a genius in adult dementias. He took thirty-three scans of children presenting with "autism" (most research studies do ten or twelve scans) and separated them as mild, moderate, or severe, and then told me what was working and not working in each instance—all without meeting a single child. That was the end of my debate regarding the validity and usefulness of these scans.

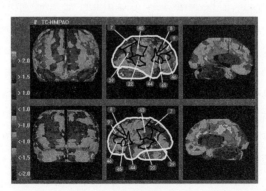

NeuroSPECT – pinpointing areas of dysfunction – a child with "autism"

Because of this early work, Dr. Mena and I had the fortunate experience of obtaining scans (eventually more than 130) on children with "autism" before they were subjected to many of the anecdotal, potentially harmful therapies being done today. These "clean" children were remarkably consistent with both the adults presenting with CFS/CFIDS and the adolescents and children now presenting with mixed and quiet ADHD. The key repetitive finding was hypoperfusion, decreased function in key areas of the temporal lobes explaining much of this dysfunction in adults and then the children, with patterns that were consistent only with a neuroimmune, disease-type process, not a metabolic or congenital disorder.

Dr. Mena also noted a phenomenon of "hyperfrontality" (increased blood flow in the frontal lobes), which was common in young children, a routine finding in the old-fashioned hyper-ADD child. It quickly became apparent that the key to "neuroimmune" was the obvious shutting down of blood flow, shutting down of function.

> This compares to what happens when a child or adult has a cold/upper respiratory infection, a virus we know does not go to the brain. We will feel "zoney," "spacey," tired, and achy. That is our immune system shutting down blood flow to key parts of the brain (the temporal lobes, limbic system, amygdala) to "protect" them. Then when we've recovered, four to seven days laters, those areas open back up, the immune system calms down, and we feel better physically and mentally.

Upon scanning adults and then children who have done many anecdotal, proposed therapies, it became very disturbing to find either diffuse areas of hypoperfusion or multiple areas of hyperperfusion in areas of the brain that had up to that time always been presenting as normal, not directly affected by this disease process itself. For me, it has been a very upsetting but striking confirmation that doing things in a random manner to the whole brain (or body), doing procedures that would never be considered physiologic in a child (or adults) not only is unlikely to help, but also has the possibility of creating additional harm or dysfunction.

NeuroSPECT: Assessment of Abnormal Distribution of Rcbf in CFIDS versus "Autistic Syndrome Children."

Michael Goldberg, Ismael Mena, Bruce. Miller, and Carmen Thomas.
Dept. of Nuclear Medicine, Imaging Center, Harbor UCLA Medical Center, Torrance, CA[36].

The study was done to compare our preliminary NeuroSPECT finding in twenty-five children diagnosed "autistic syndrome/PDD" with thirteen children previously scanned with CFS/CFIDS. This was compared to a normal database.

In the findings points that stood out were that "autistic" children often had increased blood flow in the frontal lobes (part of this may be physiologic in young children), and there were characteristically low areas of flow in the temporal and occipital lobes and cerebellum. These changes were significant compared to normals. Interesting, comparatively, the children with CFIDS also showed temporal-lobe hypoperfusion (as noted previously, a key point, the literal hallmark, of this disorder), along with decreased flow in the parietal lobes and part of the frontal lobes.

With this striking insight, it was our conclusion "that the common observation of temporal lobe hypoperfusion in adults and children with CFS/CFIDS, may define 'autism' as a disorder of impaired relations with the surrounding environment determined by the temporal hypofunction leading as a consequence to a diaschetic hypofunction of visual cortex and cerebellum." In English that means we were looking at a significant overlap of areas of dysfunction in the brain between these disorders, providing us with an objective, explainable reason for the dysfunctions being reported "mysteriously" in these children. We were looking at anatomical markings, defining autism/PDD dysfunction, correlating to models proposed by behavioral neurologists. We tried to encourage further evaluation of this phenomenon with a focus on the likely immune dysregulation that could be causing it. It was our hope that the NeuroSPECT could open the door a more physiologic/medical approach to these processes in children. Sadly that is not what has occurred.

With this research, back in 1995, I put forth at an "autistic" conference our emerging hypothesis: *Temporal lobe dysfunction is the primary source of dysfunction in many/most cases of autism, CFS/CFIDS, NIDS, and some/many cases of ADHD. The decrease in blood flow and function is secondary to immune system "activation" and/or "dysregulation".*

> With refinements and the recognition for the increased and disturbing role of a complex viral process (still with immune system primary, the virus/viruses secondary to that), the statement remains a very realistic, very logical explanation for understanding and dealing with this disaster. Why the "system" has not decided so is the enlarging mystery and ongoing disaster.

Our early work culminated in 1999 with the publication of our finding on NeuroSPECT showing the similarities and differences of the disorders being called autism, ADHD, OCD, and other neurocognitive disorders including CFS/CFIDS in adults and then children. I remain very thankful for meeting researchers like Dr. Ismael Mena, Dr. Bruce Miller, then years, now decades ahead of their time. In these various learning fields today, without documented imaging, newer ways to document and understand the differences, the confusions and potential mistakes with therapy remain abundant. With increased incidence of learning disorders comes a greater need to understand and define the dysfunction in these children by objective, "functional" quantifications.

Being exposed to the use of NeuroSPECT early opened the doors to an understanding of these evolving strange disorders called autism, ADHD, OCD, and more. In these seemingly mysterious, supposedly development-based disorders, there were similar patterns of significant frontal and temporal lobe dysfunction. Perhaps some of the misdirection, the mistakes begin made today are explainable by the ongoing lack of insight in research studies to what is really happening in the brain, what is changing or not changing with medication. Thanks to the work with NeuroSPECT, experts way beyond me were able to say early on that something was wrong, that our findings were not consistent with the ideas, the images of "autism." Early along it became obvious that in the hands of a researcher like Dr. Bruce Miller, one could understand and explain areas of the brain that were working and not working, and the dysfunctions that resulted. I wonder how we can now be in the twenty-first century and yet not demand data like this on any study regarding cognitive dysfunction and any study looking at what we call "neurotropic" agents.

The objective, "functional" quantification by NeuroSPECT offered an easy explanation for the progressive process of the autistic syndrome that occurs frequently between fifteen and twenty-four months of age. It is this immune-mediated, abnormal shutdown of blood flow in the brain that affects the language and social skills area of the brain and central nervous system function. The dysfunction/lack of blood flow can eventually lead to injury of nerve cells. This evolves into part of the explanation for the increasing number of children with abnormal brain waves and the large numbers of autistic syndrome children having concurrent seizures and epilepsy. (See the discussion on seizures.) Consistently on NeuroSPECT (in early studies, with "clean" children, those not on other therapies or remedies) we saw the following: decreased left temporal lobe function (explaining and pinpointing areas of severe speech and language dysfunction), and decreased right temporal lobe function explaining areas needed for social interaction and social integration with our environment and others. Finally (to our surprise) we repeatedly saw abnormal cerebellar involvement, explaining the appearance of so many children with usually fine and sometimes gross motor difficulties. As noted elsewhere, the issues of fine or gross motor abnormalities were not expected or discussed in the literature of the 1940s, 1950s, or 1960s, or ever noted in expected finding or criteria for autism, a major indicator that this is not the same thing.

We found autism, pervasive developmental disorder (PDD), attention deficit hyperactivity disorder (ADHD), and obsessive-compulsive disorder (OCD) involve significant frontal and temporal lobe dysfunction. This conclusion is based on NeuroSPECT work now in progress on children afflicted with these disorders. We have been using NeuroSPECT to image cerebral abnormalities of perfusion/function in autism, ADHD, OCD, and other neurocognitive disorders. With the increased focus and presentation of children labeled autistic syndrome/PDD has come a greater need to understand and define the dysfunction in these children by objective functional quantification, which is now possible with new imaging technology such as NeuroSPECT.

This offers an explanation for the process of the autistic syndrome that occurs sometime between fifteen and twenty-four months of age. The immune-mediated, abnormal shutdown of blood flow in the brain affects the language and social skills area of the brain and central nervous system function. The dysfunction caused by the lack of blood flow can eventually lead to injury of nerve cells. This is a possible explanation for the abnormal brain waves and the large numbers of autistic syndrome children suddenly being labeled as Landau-Kleffner.

We are seeing abnormal NeuroSPECT scans. There is hypoperfusion in the temporal lobes (primary dysfunction), hypoperfusion in the occipital/parietal lobes, and hypoperfusion in the cerebellum. Sadly we are finding scalloping and thinning (in some); this is actual loss of brain tissue and explains LKS and abnormal EEGs. These same children and adults have normal MRIs, and normal CAT scans.

With the NeuroSPECT, one could begin to explain various issues of learning difficulties and multiple variations of attention deficit dysfunction beginning to evolve at that time. (As noted earlier, the variations are now far more common than the classical, typical hyper-ADD child; again maybe because this has nothing to do with our original ideas of ADD/ADHD.) A key point from this work was that most of these children had normal MRIs and normal CAT scans. How can we expect to obtain new information and develop a new understanding of these disorders if we are in the twenty-first century but want to continue to use twentieth-century tools—tools, which became very good at defining the black-and-white structure of the brain, but do not give any idea of how those apparently intact areas are really functioning? Without that insight, without that understanding, this book—and the real chance to understand these mysterious disorders now, not in another decade or two—would not be possible. It is my hope that this book leads to a demand for technology application and answers now for so many children and adults with these interconnected disorders.

hed Pencils

ntries.

7

HOW EVALUATION
AND TREATMENT BEGIN:
THE GOLDBERG APPROACH

Intro to Therapy: An Overview of The Goldberg Approach

M Y BACKGROUND IN BASIC SCIENCE, CLINICAL logic, research, and the ongoing support and evolution for the idea of a complex neuroimmune, complex viral disorder / NIDS has evolved into an overall approach to therapy called The Goldberg Approach. This approach has evolved over many years and is a starting point to evaluate its application for patients with autism/ASD, ADHD, and chronic fatigue (in a more formal protocol, it can potentially create an expedited pathway to evaluate new pharmaceutical agents or other potential therapeutic choices). Until new pharmaceutical solutions evolve, this has become a multistep (similar to multiantibiotic therapy now common for ulcers) combined therapy approach.

Step one is always dietary elimination (including most nonpharmaceutical supplements). The key to helping the immune system is not how many different products and things can one throw into it, but rather how many negative stimuli (primarily foods or other non-pharmaceutically pure ingested products) you can remove from the immune system, in turn allowing the immune system the first chance to start to become healthier. While so many studies focus on the effects of pharmaceuticals, they fail to realize that food may be the biggest drug of all.

It is important to remember that since this disease did not start metabolically, you are not going to cure a patient by dietary manipulations alone, but it is a major first step to helping a child (or an adult) with these disorders (and likely many others).

The next step, dependent on lab workup and clinical history, is prescribing an antiviral for many of the patients. The antivirals are in what we call antiherpes medications. This is partly because, as presented, potential CNS herpes viruses are obviously playing a very large role in this disorder. Unfortunately, to this day, many in the research world will debate whether the proof is absolute, even though the literature and markers overwhelmingly confirm the likely presence of herpes-related viruses. These specific antivirals are also safe to administer to children because of their mode of action (they work on a metabolic point that the Herpes virus needs for survival), as long as they are monitored and dosed appropriately. Adults with Herpes remain on them their entire lives with little if any side effects. In further research trials there will be studies of stronger antiherpetic antivirals, and if indicated, potentially other types of antivirals. The key in choosing treatments for patients with this disorder is that they must be safe.

The third step is administering an antifungal (the use of antifungals is still of great debate in some medical circles because of all the misconceptions and misrepresentations). Based on work in adults and children, we know that when the immune system is stressed, something we call delayed hypersensitivity often is not working right (delayed hypersensitivity, often called tuberculin-type hypersensitivity, is our body's delayed response to a threat—a rash from poison oak or a reaction to an allergy skin test or tuberculosis skin test are all examples of how our healthy immune system is expected to react). When delayed hypersensitivity is not working correctly, since it is the key part of our immune system that handles yeast and fungal issues, there is a place for a potential yeast or fungal overgrowth in any patient. While a yeast overgrowth in theory may add to symptoms of fatigue, achiness, spaciness, and more the exact mechanism (a general GI overgrowth, interference with absorption versus possible release of a toxin) is debatable even today. Doing trials looking at markers based on the immune system—not based on blood, stool, or urine testing because of their notorious inaccuracy—there is a way to formerly evaluate and document when an excess of yeast, a yeast overgrowth, is likely. By administering antifungals to correct this overgrowth (again used correctly, chosen cautiously and monitored carefully), we can help balance another stressor to the immune system in patients.

Finally, based on clinical symptoms, and the now common denominator in these patients of temporal lobe hypoperfusion (to different degrees), comes the usage of an SSRI. This comes as step number four, since an SSRI was not originally designed to treat immune system dysfunction or viruses (if present). After diet control, antiviral, and if indicated, an antifungal, then I begin to look at using an SSRI. As explained many times to parents and patients, I do not use an SSRI, nor should trials be done, to treat a particular *symptom* (though helping temporal lobe function can help many "symptoms" seen as part of this dysfunction), especially to try to control behaviors and/or calm down or sedate a child—but because with the research and work that has evolved it is obvious that most of the *origin* of the symptoms and dysfunction is based in the temporal lobes of the brain. As confirmed repeatedly on NeuroSPECT, they are under working, under perfused— conveniently the temporal lobes are primarily serotonin mediated—it is logical to say that if you could take an agent and make the serotonin that is produced stay around longer constructively, that can and does help restore function to those areas (which in turn can address some "symptoms" but in a very physiologically healthy manner by helping restore function). And that is what SSRIs do. Unlike old-fashioned antidepressants that literally could sedate or affect the entire brain, an SSRI selectively works to block the reuptake of serotonin being produced naturally. Done judiciously and correctly, this has turned out to be an extremely important and positive step of The Goldberg Approach. This is visible and can be confirmed on repeat Spect scans, showing reversal of the low perfusion, and normalization to the areas of the brain that were not working right before therapy. One of the most dramatic presentations is that of a child (multiple children in fact; see case studies at the end of the book) who could not speak, but as their temporal lobe normalized, with good appropriate speech therapy, *the child regained speech and language function. Not just younger children, but older children too.*

The approach also encourages the role (as will be discussed) for potentially adjunctive, supportive therapies based on the individual and their particular testing or markers. Examples included usage of antibiotics for a potential strep infection, agents to help balance frontal lobe hyperperfusion such as Strattera or Wellbutrin, Tenex (often indicated for basal ganglia, lower brainstem hyperperfusion), and selectively a few others. Since the focus is children, the focus must always be on a specific need or indication, and the potential for long-term safety (or harm).

Combining the above steps of therapy, it has been my repeated pleasure to see children return to levels of function never predicted before. (As I have noted repeatedly to a happy parent, that success is expected and only possible in terms of a disease, never in a developmental disorder). While not every child is where I would like (the urgency to build and improve on The Goldberg Approach), I have many, many children not only in regular academic classes (at all grade levels), but children who are in honors, have graduated high school with honors, who are now in college. In a now healthy manner, these children are leading lives as my wife once commented *"we would all like for any of our children."* The joy of the success stories is enormous, but cannot make up for the sadness that we continue to live in a world that does not believe we are "losing" children of that potential, but that rather mistakenly subscribes to the myth of "autism." While not yet simple or easy, every child deserves this chance, every parent and family deserves a right to believe and hope. A key point, is in every patient who has stayed with me (unfortunately, especially in the early days, many parents gave up quite prematurely or did not follow diet, etc.) has done better, is a functioning member of the family, and no child with me has had to be admitted to a group home! Even when full success (a bright eyed, healthy child, functioning fully normally) is not possible, there is a tremendous ability to improve brain function, help improve health and quality of life for all. While in reality it is inevitable that our research world and scientific community will have to reach the same conclusion—that this is a treatable, medical disease—the parents meanwhile remain on the front lines with a firm focus and belief in these patients really being children that can be "returned" to their normal state.

The long-term goal of my approach is formalization and standardization of this protocol. With the use of advanced immune, genomic, NeuroSPECT, and other markers, it would become possible to accelerate a further understanding of the successes and failures of this method and thereby help expedite development of new agents and new pharmaceutical aids much faster than otherwise would occur. Opening the door to understanding what could be done, the right role for true immune modulators, could change therapy for children with these disorders, and many related disorders in adults, in a dramatically positive manner. Used correctly, chosen correctly, we can open the door to how to actually make our immune systems healthy and in turn potentially change long-term disease outcomes for many.

Patient Workup and Evaluation

Before patients are accepted into the practice, I review their records and see if they fit under the description of NIDS. Since most of the patients I see are children, they come to my office originally diagnosed with a different problem, usually autism/PDD, ADHD, or chronic fatigue syndrome. Most children I see give evidence of immune factors or viral factors. We're looking at an illness creating a dysfunction in what was previously a regular child, rather than this vague concept of something happening in utero. When you look at the data from these children, their viral markers, and the progression of their development, it becomes very obvious that one can only explain this by reference to a disease state.

To review: Somewhere between twelve, fifteen, or eighteen months (sometimes even later), these children slowly digress into this disorder labeled autism. But if you look at how the brain works, if you understand biology, you cannot have a normal child for twelve, fifteen, or eighteen months of life, a child who shows skills in developing and then loses those skills or stops progressing, and somehow try to think that something went wrong before that child was born. This is only explainable by a disease process.

Next I look for past histories supportive of immune factors in the family history, such as allergies, asthma, migraines, rheumatoid, or potential autoimmune-mediated disorders (including MS, lupus, Alzheimer's, Parkinson's, CFS, or fibromyalgia; often a major factor in parents, particularly the mother, of these children), IBS, ulcerative colitis, or Crohn's disease—in short, anything atypical.

I have to decide if the patients' charts show a pattern consistent with NIDS research. For instance, most of the children that I am seeing may be viewed as a subtype. A lot of the children I have seen have regressed and have lost skills. That means that they had words but then lost them and then did not progress. I have also seen improvements in hypotonia (low muscle tone, often previously thought untreatable) in a definite subgroup of these children. The following checklists, notes, and procedures are typical of what a parent can expect when they consult my practice for help with a child showing symptoms of autism (or any NIDS disorder).

I look at several types of medical issues that may be related to autism/NIDS, including immunologic problems.

Past history:

- ➢ Increased incidence (in mothers) of
  - • Miscarriages
  - • Infertility
  - • Preeclampsia
- ➢ Bleeding during pregnancy
- ➢ Prenatal, perinatal stress of the child

A past medical history (of conditions associated with autism in the past) needs to be ruled out

- ➢ Tuberous sclerosis (genetic)
- ➢ PKU (metabolic)
- ➢ Congenital rubella (viral)
- ➢ Down syndrome (genetic—chromosome 21)
- ➢ Fragile X (genetic)

Keys on intake:

- ➢ History of being normal until between twelve, fifteen, and eighteen months of age and then proceeding to cognitive issues and their dysfunction (often label of autism/PDD)

➤ Child with motor (fine, gross, or coordination) issues. This has become a clinical flag for a high probability of a viral component
   • Stress at intake. In the literature forty or fifty years ago, there was *no* discussion of motor abnormalities with "autism/PDD" (psychological, DSMIV category disorder); now these children routinely have motor issues

➤ History of seizures or atypical EEGs. These were *not* typical in the literature years ago. They were so rare that something called "Landau-Kleffner" was not even known by an excellent pediatric neurologist in the mid-1990s. Now we are routinely saying that 35–40 percent of these children will develop a seizure disorder. This has become an extremely strong point clinically for either a virus or a more severe autoimmune immune/vasculitis process.

Information required before the first office appointment:

Children:

➤ Complete medical history from parents, typed
➤ Medical records including neurological and psychological evaluations
➤ All prior treatments
➤ Past labs
➤ MRIs or other procedures

Adults:

➤ Medical history from onset of symptoms and before
➤ Medical records including current medications and dosages
➤ All prior treatments
➤ Past labs
➤ MRIs or other procedures

First Visit (questionnaire):

- ➢ Patient presentation, complaints, current diagnoses
- ➢ History and important items to note:
  - Birth history/trauma
  - Age of: sat alone _____, walked _____
  - Asthma
  - Eczema or hives
  - Allergies to medications
  - Convulsions
  - Tonsillitis
  - Constipation
  - Diarrhea
  - Any episode of unconsciousness
  - Temper tantrums
  - Family conflicts or problems
  - Diabetes
  - Rheumatoid arthritis in family
  - Thyroid issues in family
  - Ulcerative colitis in family
  - Migraine headaches in family
  - Asthma, eczema, or hives in family
  - Recurrent ear infections
- ➢ Current medications/treatments
- ➢ Current supplements
- ➢ Symptoms—most important items:
  - Nonrestorative sleep
  - Trouble falling asleep
  - Waking during night
  - Rash of herpes simplex or shingles
  - Fatigue
  - Memory disturbance
  - Frequently saying the wrong word
  - Depression

- Anxiety
- Panic attacks
- Headaches
- Seizures
- Ringing in ears
- Intolerance to bright lights
- Recurrent flulike illnesses
- Painful lymph nodes

➢ Severe nasal and other allergies
➢ Muscle and joint aches with trigger points or fibromyalgia
➢ Irritable bowel syndrome
➢ Low-grade fevers
➢ Night sweats
➢ Severe PMS
➢ TMJ syndrome
➢ Mitral valve prolapse
➢ Frequent canker sores
➢ Thyroid inflammation
➢ Dyspnea on exertion
➢ Multiple sensitivities to medicine, food, and other substances
➢ Problems during pregnancy
➢ Maternal fever
➢ Maternal bleeding
➢ Perinatal bleeding
➢ Perinatal or neonatal asphyxia
➢ Neonatal infection
➢ Maternal miscarriages
➢ Autoimmune disease
➢ Rheumatoid disease
➢ Lupus
➢ Normal developmental milestones, then changes
➢ Frequent ear infections
➢ Asthma

- Hay fever
- Eczema
- Migraines
- Constipation
- Diarrhea
- Hospitalizations
- Obsessive compulsive tendencies
- Lethargy
- Staring spells
- "Tuned out"
- Muscle tone
- Coordination
- Motor skills, fine and gross
- Focus/attention
- Spaciness
- Speech/verbalization
- Hyper
- Socialization
- Appetite
- Eye contact
- What type of educational setting? Special education, regular classroom, shadow in class, etc.

Review paperwork
Review commitment to care and weekly update procedure
Explain SPECT scan, referral
Explain and order blood work
Discuss diet/elimination
Perform basic health exam—HR, BP, Ht, Wt, BS, HEENT, chest, heart, abdomen, extremities, and basic neuro.
Baseline neuropsych test? (when in formal protocols)

Questions asked at each office visit, by the admitting nurse:

Children:

- ➢ What medications and doses are currently being used?
- ➢ What does the patient's diet consist of?
- ➢ Is child spacey or zoney?
- ➢ How is the child's sleep cycle?
- ➢ Is the child waking rested, or tired?
- ➢ Has the child been hyper or aggressive?
- ➢ How is the child doing academically?
- ➢ How are the child's social interactions?
- ➢ Does the child initiate play?
- ➢ Is the child interested in play?
- ➢ How is the child's appetite?
- ➢ Does the child crave or want any one particular food?
- ➢ Does the child have any allergy or cold symptoms?
- ➢ What has changed positive/negative since the last visit
  - Particularly related to medication changes that may have occurred
- ➢ Any pickup in language or skills?
- ➢ What supplements (if any) is the child currently taking?

Adults:

- ➢ What medications and doses are currently being used?
- ➢ What supplements are you currently taking?
- ➢ What does the patient's diet consist of?
- ➢ How is your sleep cycle?
- ➢ Are you waking rested?
- ➢ Do you have any brain fog or memory problems?
- ➢ Do you have any muscle or joint pain?
- ➢ How is your cognition?
- ➢ How is your appetite?
- ➢ Any sensitivity to light?

Appointment procedure completed by the physician:

> ➢ Medical evaluation: breath sounds, heart rate, visual inspection of EENT
> ➢ Consult about patient/caregiver responsibility for treatment
> ➢ Order for SPECT scan? (depending upon clinical protocol)
> ➢ Order for blood work if determined necessary; may include any or all of the following:

CBC (with full manual differential)

Sedimentation rate

CMV IgG/IgM

ANA titer

EBV IgG/IgM

Hypothyroid panel

Ferritin level

Immune panel—	Total & % CD4
	Total & % CD8
	Total & % CD16/CD56
	Total & % CD19

Lead level (if never done)

Vitamin B12 level

Folic acid

Vitamin A level (if history of supplements)

Vitamin D level (if never done, or on supplements)

Comprehensive metabolic panel

Lipid panel

HHV6 titer IgG/IgM

Quantitative immunoglobulins (IgG, IgA, IgM, IgE)

Gliadin antibodies IgG/IgA

ASO titer

Alpha interferon (very optional expensewise)

HSV I/II—IgG/IgM

Allergy food screen (IgG4 based ninety-five foods)

➢ I may or may not need to prescribe antibiotics to handle issues of bronchitis, ear infections, or strep throat.

➢ Any time a medication is prescribed or a dosage changed, the patient is informed of what response is intended and what reactions, both good and bad, to be aware of, and when to call the office if there are negative reactions.

Note: My office has the capability to do rapid strep tests, tympanograms, and other quick diagnostics. I belong to a nationally certified lab that does routine blood work as well as immune testing.

(Note: Regular follow-ups, updates, and controlling changes are critical to understanding a patient—child or adult—and coming to the best answers and choices for that individual)

Weekly Updates:

Patients are required to submit weekly information updates via fax or e-mail and include:

➢ Date
➢ Patient Name
➢ Patient Date of Birth
➢ Patient Weight
➢ Current Medications and Dosages
➢ Date of Recent Dosage Change
➢ Positives (especially in relationship to any recent medication change)
➢ Negatives (especially in relationship to any recent medication change)
➢ Comments

Second Visit:

Review SPECT (if done) and blood work findings
Review confirm diet changes

Basic health exam
Prescribe meds if indicated

or

Monthly Telephone Consultations:
(For those not within driving distance)

Patients have a monthly twenty- to forty-minute telephone consultation with me. I access the patients' computer charts, review the previous patient treatment and recent weekly updates, and query the patients (or the patients' parents) as to their present health and brain function. I add new patient health information and medication and dosage changes directly to the patients' computer charts. My telephone consultation questions and treatment changes/additions are based on the conversation with the patients and the patients' previous treatment and blood work results documented on the computer chart. It is the same as if you were standing in front of me, except for the acute physical exam. (I request parents see their local physician if there are any issues of acute or unexplained illness suspected.)

Subsequent Visits:
- Confirm compliance with medication, diet, and weekly updates
- Detailed update (supplementing weekly updates) regarding any changes related to medication changes (good or bad) along with, at the time of the visit, details regarding overall progress, brightness, dullness, the child's sense of being connected and receptive to learning, and difficulties arising from behavior or learning techniques and backgrounds.
- Review most recent blood work, order additional if needed
- Basic health exam
- Adjust medications per protocol and patient's condition
- Check need for consultations with other care providers on progress
- Six months and/or one year: Order NeuroSPECT (if indicated)

- Neuropsych testing or "wellness" quotient updated (with any formal study)
- Any changes at all either positive or negative (there should be no ongoing negatives!)
- One should monitor complete blood count (CBC) with differential, and a chemistry panel (focusing on liver functions and kidney functions) on any child using a pharmaceutical medication of any kind at least bimonthly (initially on protocol—first year may be monthly)

  Having many children (and adults) on antivirals from three to four months, often one to two years, many now much longer. I will always show routine monitoring (which should help to support safety over this long-term)

  • Only significant toxicity issue appears to be kidney function (*only* transient in one or two children over all these years)
- Would advise monitoring growth and development (done on some of the patients; if a retrospective or prospective study is pursued, it would likely be available around the country by their physicians).

  • Confirmed by general good height, often better growth (recovering from illness), but may have weight issue (variable)

Patient Blood work

Lab test	High value	Low value	Normal	Considerations
Allergens, food				
ANA				
ASO titer				
B 12 and folate				
CBC with diff and plt				
Celiac screen – Gliadin antibodies				
CMV IgG/IgM				
Comprehensive metabolic panel				
EBV series				
HHV-6				
HSV				
IgG subclasses				
Immunoglobulins, quant.				
Lipid panel				
Sedimentation rate				
Super Panel—iron, ferritin, TIBC				
T & B lympho-cytes/NK cells				
Thyroid antibodies				
TSH, sensitive				

Background

As a physician with a strong background in what we call basic sciences (college and medical school) and then a strong clinical and research exposure heavy on immunology, infectious disease, allergies, and endocrinology, I watched these patterns of illness and diseases change before my eyes (less than a decade in practice). It was rapidly obvious that the only likely common denominator was the immune system. We study all kinds of environmental stresses and exposures, immune markers, and variations of multiple immune-related diseases without ever stepping back and realizing the real key is the immune system itself.

The disorders discussed in this book (and other related ones) can begin to be corrected—the key is having a healthy functioning immune system. Any effort to push the system one way or the other is going to create a problem, cause extra stress on the system, and could lead to further harm.

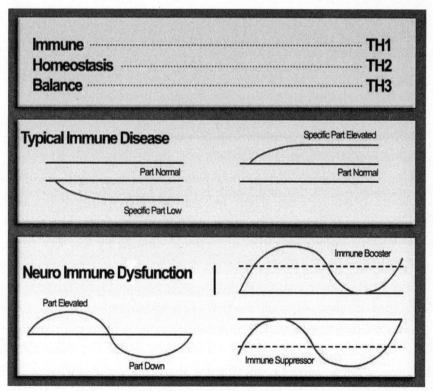

IMMUNE SYSTEM—ACTIVATED/SUPPRESSED VERSUS DYSFUNCTIONAL

Some of these children over the years have had positive ANA (antinuclear antibody) titers—a classical marker for the potential of lupus or other autoimmune disease. This is ignored in children diagnosed with autism. The argument is that we are merely detecting positive ANAs more often with better techniques and that it does not signify any other problems within these children. The problem with that reasoning is that if in training I was taught a positive ANA was not good—was the harbinger for potentially bad things—then just because we have better lab techniques, what makes it okay to dismiss now "at low levels," much less when there are significantly elevated ones. A positive ANA means the body is making antibodies against the nucleus of its own cells. At any level, any degree, how can this be okay, how can this not be potentially pathologic in these children, any positive child or adult?

> Contrary to general medical teaching, I have seen many positive ANAs turn negative, once an immune system is given a chance to return to normal—by removing ongoing stressors with The Goldberg Approach. This does not involve using steroids or other strong, potentially harmful, immune suppressant agents.

Before approaching therapy in a patient, one must understand the patient and their illness, their whole body and how it is creating dysfunction, and what those dysfunctions really are. As a physician, as a clinician, I was given a unique insight into this "mysterious" disorder by first working as noted with my wife and then some other mothers in the practice presenting with this new, "mysterious" illness in adults being called CFS/CFIDS. The insight into the clinical dysfunction of these children was sadly all too easy to connect after working with adults and teenagers who could remember when they functioned normally and who could remember and relate to what was working and not working for them presently and before the illness. What can this be like for a child who has no "well" perspective to relate to? If not previously damaged, or miswired "mysteriously," how much are these children being left to suffer?

Think about the comparison in adults and children and the real overlap of symptoms and problems occurring in both. For adults (often previously high-functioning, type A, college-educated people) with CFS/CFIDS it is common to have severe sleep problems, classically what we call a "nonrestorative" sleep cycle. In the mid-1980s I was exposed to research documenting that these supposedly "psychosomatic" adults had an altered stage IV, REM sleep cycle. This explained how an adult (and now these children) can sleep for hours yet wake up mentally and physically still tired. Likewise, adults with CFS/CFIDS often would report "sensitivity to bright lights." Many of these children have the same obvious symptom. In an excellent medical school, with excellent professors, I was taught "sensitivity to bright lights" meant inflammation or "a virus on the brain" till proven otherwise. Shouldn't those patients, both children and adults, receive that same scrutiny, that same concern, today? These children may not only have sensitivity to bright lights but also may exhibit intolerance to heat (just like lupus patients or others with "autoimmune"-mediated disorders).

Consider that when this disease, which we are calling NIDS, affects a previously intelligent, usually high-functioning adult, they will now have distressing memory and concentration loss, word blocking, fogginess, forgetfulness. They are overwhelmed by loud and conflicting noises, have impaired judgment, and are unable to link up auditory and visual input. They may develop dyslexic-like symptoms, have difficulty maintaining attention set, and often will have difficulties/impairment in inputting, encoding, and retrieving information (comprehending and remembering what has been read).

If these dysfunctions can occur with a mature adult brain, it is not hard to understand (especially thanks to NeuroSPECT) how a supposedly "autistic" child will present with abnormal responses to sensations—often a combination of sight, hearing, touch, pain, balance, smell, and taste. The way a child holds his body will be affected; there will be disturbances in the rate of appearance of physical, social, and language skills (to the extent speech and language are frequently absent or delayed); and there will be altered thinking, abnormal ways of relating to people, objects, and events. This is essentially the same process that we witness in adults, but an immature brain in a child.

Author Note: These related changes have been documented repeatedly with adults, with the medical literature over thirty years ago demonstrating outright development of "autistic" symptoms, in a previously normal individual from a herpes virus. How much longer are we going to ignore the obvious? We're ignoring the fact that these children are suffering from a real disease, not an impossible, "mysterious" presumed neurodevelopmental disorder.

Role of Diet Elimination and Reduction of Allergy-Related Stresses

To constructively begin to approach therapy and ultimately prevention in these children, one must start with a background that is versed in an understanding of the physiology and the biology of children. As noted, I remain thankful for my medical and residency training, which resulted in an early exposure to collagen vascular disorders (the principles behind many autoimmune disorders today), along with a heavy emphasis on infectious disease, immunology, and allergies. A professor (many years ahead of his time) taught me to consider the role of food in creating stress and the subsequent reactions within the immune system.

With the first step of therapy being the removal of triggers that create ongoing stress to a child, the next step for me as a pediatrician becomes how I can apply my medical school training, my postgraduate training, and new tools and information that have evolved since to help a child further reduce stresses and the dysfunction within the body in order to help the immune system and brain become healthy. This would not be possible with *developmental* autism/PDD, ADHD, etc., but it is expected and very possible when these disorders are recognized as variations of a disease process.

The idea of removing dairy was not always an accepted practice. It has been a sad point for medicine that if we cannot conclusively document or prove with markers what is happening to the body, the medical profession is all too quick to dismiss it. I had professors who taught me to think, question, understand, and be skeptical. Sadly we have entered an era of medicine in which you do A, B, C, and D, but if you do not respond to ABCD, you are often out of luck or considered to be psychosomatic. We are in a world in which the general pediatrician has to be very cautious, very afraid of doing anything not dictated as correct by the AAP or his or her local medical society.

It may seem like common sense, but I was taught if a child was chronically congested or having upset stomachs, rashes, eczema, or allergy symptoms, take away potential triggers. Don't just keep treating the symptoms, the recurrent ear infections, the bronchitis, and so forth. The teaching in this country was that colic was merely evidence of a child's immature brain or immature system and was therefore unavoidable.

However Europeans generally believe colic does originate from the GI tract, and they believe strongly in the connection with the stomach. Because I recommended preventive diets, taking children off dairy, and avoiding exposure to allergenic foods and substances, very few children in my regular practice suffered from colic, chronic rashes, eczema, etc. We must understand that a baby's superreactive GI sensitivity is a strong background and great training and experience for the GI sensitivity affecting so many children and adults today. The best way to help a stomach do better and relieve stress was not to gauge how many things I could throw into it, but, rather, to focus on *removing the negatives.*

All of these children (and adults with these disorders) have superreactive GI tracts. When a mother asks, "What is the best thing to give my child to help his immune system?" my response is always, "Take away the negatives."

Much of my background comes from my training as a pediatrician, looking at babies as having very sensitive GI tracts. If there was ever an understanding, an on-the-job "induction" preparing me for these children now, it was certainly and thankfully my training. Thinking about what impact foods have on the stomach of a baby, and being trained always to introduce foods very slowly, and not to introduce solids too soon to a child, I have great skepticism. I tend to be concerned what may be firing off the child's stomach, their immune system. Early along I learned that if I gave whole-grain, "natural" and "healthy" food to young babies, it often sent them up the wall. The principle is clear: Nothing can be healthy for an adult or child if it fires off the GI tract and the immune system.

I began telling mothers they should avoid dairy and whole grains (and other allergenic foods) during pregnancy. While breast feeding is good, I advised pregnant women and new mothers to stay off dairy, whole grains, and other allergic foods if she was going to be breast feeding. While we believe nursing is in theory better for a child, we seem to forget that anything a mother eats can go through her breast milk. Whether a mother was nursing or making sure formula choices were not causing GI irritability, congestion, and rashes, this led to a generally very healthy pediatric practice and is the starting point for preventing stress in children being born today. Since, over the years I always practiced preventative pediactric medicine, I found myself first focusing on feeding and nursing advice to prevent allergies and congestion in infants and children. Also, consistent now with recommendations from the Academy of Pediatrics I practice allergy prevention and stress management with pregnant mothers—preventative care in the womb. While my first focus was mothers within my practice getting ready to have their next child this also involved preventative advice for any parent with a history of allergies or immune disorders in their families, or who had a previous child who showed symptoms of NIDS.

Working with babies was yet another learning lesson. A child might tolerate a heat-treated, sterilized formula but react when given milk or dairy. By heat treating and processing, you change the protein structure, the allergy potential of a food. With the push to everything "natural," we are ignoring the fact that "natural" often causes allergic reactions in these children. A simple test that can be done on any child is what we call a CBC with a *full* differential that shows what are called eosinophils. If a baby has elevated eosinophils, it is a sure thing that something that child is receiving is allergenic to that child and creating immune stress. (Note: The opposite is not always true, since some children will show elevated eosinophils, but others may not—part of how imperfect lab testing for allergies can be.)

An additional learning lesson is that to avoid slip-ups, rigidity of restrictions is far more important now than it was in my early days of practice given the known role of the accumulation of stress on a fetus or infant. With the recognition a number of years ago that "bovine protein" could act as a superantigen (and trigger multiple immune reactions in an immune-sensitive individual), the Academy of Pediatrics made the recommendation that in a family with a history of atopy (that's a polite word for allergies), the mother should avoid dairy and whole-wheat foods during her pregnancy. As noted above, they missed a critical point when they did not carry that through to a mother nursing. Finally, the academy now does recommend that when there is a history of allergies in the family, a mother should avoid milk and dairy and whole-wheat whole grains when nursing. I would certainly expand that to include avoidance of red things such as strawberries, cherries, and, in this physician's experience, tropical fruits (think of what is native to where you grew up; what is not native is likely to be more difficult to handle) and with preventive caution for any food that falls into a category of potentially reactive substances. Removal of potential triggers is a key to being preventive during pregnancy, after delivery, and with the eventual slow introduction of different foods for a baby.

Sugar, dairy, and dueling dietary theories

Unfortunately, over the years, the role of diet and the need to avoid "negatives" has increased, rather than diminished. The issue of "cheating" by feeding a patient something allergenic, or cheating by giving sugars or carbohydrates, now has begun to overlap. It was always easy to say that a "cheat" with dairy or a food that was an allergen was far more disruptive than a cheat just with "sugar," but parents have often not understood that.

While sugar, or carbs (simples carbs become "sugar" in one metabolic step in the body) give an immediate "rush," can create a sugar "high" or contribute to a rebound hypoglycemia (episode of low blood sugar), an "allergic" cheat will throw off the immune system for up to seven to ten days. Worth avoiding, when thinking of long-term recovery, and the need for the body to have a chance to build itself back up, to recover. Uniquely, dairy, what we call "bovine" protein, acting as what we call a "superantigen," can set up the immune system in a dysfunctional manner, resulting (like the aftereffect of some viruses, particularly flu viruses) in the immune system attacking and wiping out the beta cells (the cell that produces insulin) in the pancreas, leaving a "predisposed" individual now diabetic, requiring shots of insulin for the rest of his or her life.

> Taking the time to explain this connection helps parents understand why diet is important, and over the years is very helpful with a child who is doing better and thinking well enough to get into "trouble." A strong reason is often better than just a vague "it can hurt you!"

The issue with carbohydrates—besides the issue of simple ones becoming sugars very easily—is that any product made from a grain, as noted elsewhere, is potentially allergenic. I will usually see ongoing "allergenic shiners" (circles under the eyes) frequently, or an elevation in what are called "basophils," as indicators for suspicion of "too many carbs," or evidence that the wrong food choices are still being made.

The role of diet is major in thinking of removal of potential triggers, in looking at how you cool down an overall reactive, inappropriately reactive immune system. Since this did not begin metabolically, and was never caused by any specific food or vitamin deficiency, one cannot expect to cure this or fix it by diet alone; but understanding the relationship between the brain, the immune system, and the gut is a key part in learning to take stresses off a child, both in treatment and prevention.

In medical school we are taught that we all have what is called a triad, a strong connection between the brain, the immune system, and the gut. Short of the immune system, the GI tract has more lymphocytes than any other organ in the body. We do not routinely think about this, but physiologically the inside of the GI tract from the mouth to the rectum is essentially outside the body. Nature designed us logically. The GI tract is lined with all these lymph cells to protect us, to prevent infection and disease. Foods and other exposures can cause tremendous reactivity that may seem to originate in the GI tract, but it is a large mistake to think this is the origin or control point of the ongoing dysfunction. It is very foolish to think that the gut would be the control point. The key, the overall control is in the brain and what we have learned is a very complex "neuroimmune" system.

As expressed earlier in the book, the neuroimmune system, not the gut, is the key to understanding this dysfunction. The neuroimmune system is in control. For example, a cold is a virus that does not go to the brain. In trying to protect us (how the system was designed), the neuroimmune system shuts down blood flow to key parts of our brain. We will feel "zoney," "spacey," tired, or achy, but in a healthy person, once well, the system returns to normal, the brain opens up again, and we feel fine and think well. If we start thinking about the shutdown going on in the children's brain, rather than many supplements and foods helping them to get better, if any food, any supplement, any product irritates the GI tract, it stimulates the immune system, leading to greater attack and shutdown of the brain. This leads back to the discussion above; the best principle to help the brain and the GI tract is removal of triggers, removal of negative exposures. The practice of removing exposures has served me extremely well over the years, both in therapy as well as in prevention.

As I found out early along, work done in the 1930s and 1940s showed that nonprescription grade products did not make it past the liver. While making most of them a waste of money, that fact may also protect some of these children from the potentially negative manipulative megadose effects.

I cannot stress enough that years of exposure and experience have taught me that the safest thing about most products that you buy in a health food store that are not pure is the body does not absorb them. It seemed at least a fairly sophisticated approach from a nutritional direction to work with a company and using prescription grade products, based on a very logical principle of doing a blood profile of amino acids, then prescribing a supplement pattern meant to help.

I soon found out that while I could often help a patient, I was not going to end this process. Believing in a strong supportive role for nutrition choices (particularly avoidance of negatives), I could help, but not solve this problem by nutrition (since it did not begin metabolically). I also learned rapidly, while trying to do things with a somewhat controlled environment, that while within the amino acids, lysine and arginine were the markers for the immune system, and most of these patients were low in one or both; it became apparent by watching and controlling individual factors that I might give a patient lysine and it might help them, but even though the body was low in arginine, if I gave arginine (which is in many of the "customized" formulas given to these children), the patient often did much worse. This was a rapid learning lesson (which ultimately made sense) that these herpes-related viruses thrived on arginine. Part of the lesson learned was that we as physicians and therapists have to be careful to not just assume the body being low in some factor is bad. The immune system may allow the reduction of arginine levels as a protective step.

A general pediatric note is needed here. Between multiple sensitivities and dietary or other manipulations, many of these children will go through periods of constipation. Always speak with your pediatrician, but over the years, I remain thankful that my pediatric GI professor was one of the top three pediatric GI specialists in the country. Over the years, physiology and basic principles again hold true. One does not want to use stimulants or laxatives (sometimes necessary under very limited circumstances, never over the long-term), but rather you must try to create a natural softening effect, then let the bowel (and the child) retrain themselves. For this purpose old-fashioned mineral oil is still an excellent choice, while if a child is old enough (too young is dangerous—can choke), I prefer something like a sugar-free Citrucel, a very safe, very natural stool softner, no laxative or stimulant effect. Since a product like "sugar-free Citrucel" is not absorbed, it is then safe over the long-term, and arguably can help regulate both constipation and diarrhea with IBS. Both types of softeners are more effective when given twice a day, amount per dosing based on child's weight and sensitivity to effect. With mineral oil, one "titrates" that the stool is soft, but ideally not oily or leaking oil. It is wise to give vitamins and most medicines at least an hour before or after administering mineral oil.

The next steps in therapy are based on attempting to use pharmaceutical agents and targeted therapies to help remove and control stresses on the immune system and the brain, and to help support restorative (not behavioral control) function for the brain, particularly the temporal lobes. As a pediatrician, I would stress the goal is a bright, alert, healthy growing child. The use of a medication (or any agent) has to be with an expectation of not only not creating harm but also helping the patient to get better, achieving and reaching healthy, potentially normal functioning. I frequently note to parents, "I am not a psychiatrist." I will not prescribe medications such as antipsychotics to "control" these children; I do not believe in them.

I will paraphrase all this by saying I look at these children as potentially healthy children fighting a serious illness, and that always brings me back to basic pediatric training and medical training: "Do no harm." As much as I want to help a child get well and win this battle and help parents who are desperate to help their child, a key restriction over the years is I cannot use a product that I know could be likely to cause harm or long-term damage to that child's body or brain. A very large mistake made while treating these children as though they have "autism" is the assumption that the child's brain is already injured or damaged. Many therapies are mistakenly applied. The use of supplements and many procedures (chelation, HBOT) may damage a child's brain. Antipsychotics or other medications could never be healthy for a potentially normal brain; because these children are sadly not considered to have normal brains, doctors and parents are willing to take risks that are otherwise unacceptable. I will always stress that the guiding principle in treatment is an expectation that the child started off with a normal or above-normal potential, and I must try to give that child a chance to recover, to be normal or above!

Antivirals

When a child starts on an antiviral, there's about 70 to 80 percent chance I'm going to get a positive response. With a positive response (often after a die-off or kill-off effect), a child on the antiviral will brighten up, become more alert, and begin to process better. If I take them off (something I do only slowly, and with great caution), and they are not in full control of the virus, they become dull and "spacey" again. In theory, the only thing you can treat with Valtrex or Famvri is a herpes-related virus. Antivirals are not neurotropic agents and don't, in theory, work on the brain. The use of an antiviral and a positive effect clinically simply helps confirm that viruses (or, at minimum, a dysfunction connected to them) are involved.

Strong lab markers supporting the likelihood of a virus are:

➤ Low NK cells (less than 4–5 percent), with or without elevated HHV6 titer.

➤ Elevated alpha interferon (should be a marker for potential viral activation for any immunologist or infectious disease specialist).

➤ Elevated HHV6 titer (40 or above Elisa, "old" titer of 1:320/ likely 1:160) or positive IgM of any of other viral screens above. In theory this only tests for one of a family (HHV6, HHV7, HHV8, and even 9 and 10 are now being detected) of viruses capable of "reactivation." (New data may be showing viral reactivation behind supposedly false elevated EBV and CMV.)

➤ Low QIgM.

- Should be suspicious of high or low QIgM as marker of a stressed immune system—low seems more typical of a possible virus.

- While not proving anything, years ago an elevated QIgM meant you looked for leukemia, lymphoma, etc., in an adult.
➢ History of fine or gross motor abnormalities or photosensitivity.
  - Years ago, photosensitivity implied viral infection and/or brain inflammation until proven otherwise. Many of these children (and adults) will have this very significant complaint, and it is ignored.
➢ History of accompanying seizure disorder or abnormal EEG.
  - As discussed, based on lack of associated seizures for many decades in discussions of autism, when this occurs one should be very suspicious about possible viral irritation, irritable foci.
➢ History of regression.

The key principle remains that a healthy immune system is our best defense against viruses, retroviruses, and multiple other potential pathogens or opportunistic organisms. Returning our immune system to healthy, normal function is going to be the key for many interrelated autoimmune, complex neuroimmune, and complex viral disorders. Currently, what I do with The Goldberg Approach is to attack with combined steps, with the goal of both reducing the stresses and removing the stresses attacking the body and the brain. With the now-consistent goal of taking stress off the immune system, trying to give the immune system a chance to become healthier, it would be a major plus to have agents that could more actively help adjust the immune system to a healthier state. It has been my goal, ever since I was exposed to information regarding a new kind of true "immune-modulator," to create a focus, create an effort to bring these rapidly into development for these disorders, and potentially many other disorders with "autoimmune" or "neuroimmune" components. Unlike all past efforts, the key is not going to be to regulate or push the immune system in one direction or the other, but rather in a very unique manner (reminiscent of nature and a mother's pregnancy) to help restore a healthy balance to the immune system.

Now the herpes virus family (including CMV—cytomegalovirus, EBV—Epstein-Barr virus, and HZV—chicken pox) is a fascinating one. In medical school when we were taught about herpes simplex (cold sores, vaginal sores), we learned if these viruses went to the brain, you were going to be very ill, or comatose—you could die in a short amount of time. The herpes virus is one of the only viruses that we call DNA-based. Most viruses are what we call RNA viruses. They live and use the cytoplasm of our cells to replicate and survive. Herpes viruses use and live within the DNA, the nucleus of our cells (particularly brain tissue, but also heart, liver, and kidney tissue). This puts these viruses in an entirely different category. In theory these viruses are known to affect our genes and chromosomes and can cause mutations.

With early viral therapy beginning to be directed at these herpes viruses, what seems to be occurring in these children and adults with these disorders is a much more chronic herpes-related infection, far more consistent with what we have learned about a family of what we now call "higher-order herpes viruses"—HHV6, HHV7, and HHV8, and the newly identified 9 and 10. The problem is these are much more sophisticated viruses. They go to the brain, but try to live low-grade. Think of this as stealth, or living below the radar. They want to live off the brain, but not upset the host so much that the immune system tries to kill them or kills the host. Herpes simplex is a very inefficient virus; you kill the host, and you kill yourself, the virus. These higher-order viruses are smarter: let's keep the host alive, and let's keep ourselves (the viruses) alive. I have never been exposed to any medical research indicating that a virus living on my brain, particularly within the temporal lobes, is going to be good for me or anyone.

With the work emerging from research on chronic fatigue syndrome in adults, one has to be open to the fact that we may be looking at some type of CMV or Epstein-Barr variant/mutation (rather than just the past concept that elevated Epstein-Barr titers and elevated CMV titers were not real, or just false activations of the immune system). The key is all of these viruses are within the herpes family of viruses, which in a backward sense may be fortuitous, because the way they behave, the way herpes simplex acted, spurred research and development of agents to try to slow down or stop these viruses. While the initial antiviral agents were potentially dangerous or not that effective, there is now a series of agents that, when monitored and dosed correctly, are considered very safe in treatment, generally speaking. This is explainable because the agents work on a mechanism that the herpes virus uses and our human bodies do not use. At the same time, there are certainly stronger, potentially more effective antiviral agents, but they do carry some risk, which I feel is not justified in children. However new, controlled, appropriate trials may be justified to look at them in the future. Presently, doing things very cautiously, I feel limited to the choices of Acyclovir (Zovirax), Valtrex, or Famvir. Contrary to misinformation, these agents are not toxic to the liver, but you do have to watch appropriately and monitor kidney function (which is easy to do with a routine chem panel—what includes a BUN and creatinine). As noted, when one looks at the role of herpes viruses, not only do they go to the brain and the CNS (central nervous system), particularly the temporal lobes, but we now know they also will go to the heart and to the liver, and there is now evidence of passage in kidney transplants. It has been my overwhelming clinical experience, while doing close liver and kidney monitoring, that when these children have liver functions mild or very moderately elevated, it is not because of a medication I may be using, but rather because of a background virus. In fact, it has been my experience, and is certainly not a surprise, that even a cold virus causes stress that can result in mild liver function elevation when a child is just normally sick. When a true toxicity or major viral infection (i.e., hepatitis-related viruses) occurs, the liver functions often will go quite high, significantly above what seems to be common in many of these children. While carefully following liver and kidney functions to document and monitor safety of any agent I will use or prescribe, it has been interesting to note that many of these children will present with "low-grade" liver elevations (often noted but ignored on past tests), in my experience, reflecting a marker for the likelihood of HHV-6 or some other herpes-related virus directly stressing the liver. It has become obvious that rather than the use of pharmaceutical agents causing more stress, by suppressing and trying to stop the virus, one removes stress from the liver (also the brain, potentially the heart). Under the guise of "autism" as physicians the "system" has essentially observed this essentially slow chronic deterioration of the brain, and often physical condition of the patient. Recognized as it should, recognized as NIDS, a medical epidemic, physicians would be expected not to let this continue to happen.

> In the early days of this, with good researchers questioning whether the antiviral treatments worked and were indicated, I would start a child on an antiviral, then watch them become brighter, sharper, better connected, then with initial success stop the antiviral, often to see many children begin to fall backward. While I would never approach weaning of an antiviral in this manner today (I do not want to allow any fallback with inadvertent reactivation), this did at the time help convince good researchers that whatever was there, whatever I was treating had to be herpes related!

Recent research

Detection of an infectious retrovirus, XMRV, in blood cells of patients with chronic fatigue syndrome (*Science* [New York, N.Y.] 2009 Oct 23;326[5952]:585–9. Epub 2009 Oct 8), showing the issue of a retrovirus in adults with chronic fatigue syndrome and a potential finding in these children labeled "autistic" only heightens the issues of viral activation, immune reactivity, and what we have learned from the study of HIV as "neuroimmune inflammation." The discussions have already begun: how many other retroviruses may be involved with this disorder, or other complex immune disorders. This has emphasized the urgency of understanding and recognizing what is a disease process in these children (as well as the adults) and rapidly attempting to develop more targeted therapies to help.

While it's safe to say most children with the aforementioned symptoms are going to be exhibiting neuroimmune dysfunction, not every child is going to have an active virus. When a child has fine or gross motor issues, has had regression in behaviors and skills, has a seizure, or has an abnormal

EEG, the likelihood of a virus, particular a herpes-related virus, being present is extremely high.

When approaching therapy for these chronic viruses, it is very obviously consistent with medical school teaching that an antibacterial agent, an antiviral, cannot be expected to do the whole job; one must have immune system help. If you are using an antiviral at correct therapeutic levels and not controlling immune reactivity and the ongoing stresses on the system, the chances that the body will be able to take control of the virus are very low. You may slow it up, you may suppress the virus, but you're not ultimately winning the fight; you will not be able then to do without the antiviral until that body can take control.

This principle is consistent with medical school teaching, illustrated by an example that in an era that an organism called pneumococcus (now a very resistant bacterial infection) was so sensitive to penicillin that the joke was you could breathe penicillin and the organism would die; yet even then, a black child was still at risk for severe septic complications, particularly of the hip and bones. This occurred because that child's immune system, due to a genetic issue, was not handling that organism correctly. This same principle applies to the issue in infectious disease many times over, and in particular applies to these children. If you're going to use a medication, you must also work to have the immune system helping, becoming an ally, part of a battle for control, restoration of balance, and health. It is important to emphasize that the use of antivirals and choice is based on a combination as discussed of safety and efficacy. If someone was in a hospital, with an overwhelming infection with CMV, HHV-6, or other serious herpes virus, one would turn to newer, stronger, potentially more toxic antiviral agents. In these children (and adults), one is not dealing with an overwhelming acute infection; instead it has a much more slow, insidious, and chronic nature. The key for now is using safe antivirals to try to suppress the virus, allowing the patient's own immune system a better chance to gain control.

Based on these steps, we are beginning to implement what we call The Goldberg Approach to avoid the mistakes being made by many. Inconsistent with good infectious disease principles, many physicians advising parents and saying they know how to treat this disorder will start and stop antivirals and/or antifungals without using blood tests to accurately monitor what they are doing, in fact whether they are even succeeding in their goals. When an antiviral is needed, you need to monitor the patient to make sure that ultimately you are getting suppression of the elevated titers (when they are present as markers), restoration of low WBCs (a common issue with these chronic viral infections), and restoration of NK cell function. To do this realistically requires a combination of working to help the immune system become healthier, clearing up the diet, and using the antiviral. It has been my experience over many years that I can reach a point where the virus may be inactive, but the immune system is not yet strong enough to take over the full job if I withdraw the antiviral. In the early days, when titers and immune systems seemed better, I would stop the antiviral. Unfortunately many of those children would then regress back into their "fog," with evidence of viral reactivation occurring. Therefore, I no longer do that. Instead, when titers are down and the immune system and the child seem healthy, I will wean down the antiviral, carefully monitoring for signs of reactivation of problems from doing that. If everything stays good, then some children certainly can come off the antiviral. Realistically this is not a short course of therapy, but just like bacteria, these viruses are becoming more resistant due to the multiple, ineffective, misuse of antivirals. These short courses, which may often "stir up" these slow viruses, are potentially just as harmful, and likely even more harmful, than not treating at all.

When you are going to try and help the body and brain become healthy, the key is nature, our own built-in defense, the immune system. When healthy, the immune system is the component that can handle viruses and even retroviruses (in theory we all have some in our bodies, but we control them, keeping them dormant or inactive when our immune systems are healthy). Ironically much of this ability is tied in to our NK cell system, the same system that protects children and adults from cancer and other serious disorders. This physician believes the major rise in childhood and adult cancers over the last decades, often in younger individuals, is likely related to this same concept of NIDS, with more and more "neurotypical" children and adults walking around in a stressed immune state. It turns out the NK (natural killer) cells are being directly attacked by the XMRV retrovirus (and most likely other yet undefined viruses as well). The more we learn, the more obvious it is becoming that perhaps the only way to really stop the "cancer epidemic," to lower significantly the cost and stresses on our medical system and families, is to come back to logic, common sense. Let's start looking at how children and adults can have healthier immune systems again. Thankfully my pediatric training was focused on preventive medicine. Over the years I would frequently tell a parent that the goal of therapy was not to save their child with a serious complication in an intensive care unit; rather, the real goal was not to have the child in the hospital at all.

> ➤ Antivirals:

Valtrex
> ➤ 1 gm tid (for adult 70 kg or above)
> > ➤ Proportion based on child's weight.
> > > ➤ i.e., 250 tid for 35 lb, 500 tid for 70 lb, etc.

or

Famvir
> ➤ 500 mg tid for 70 kg adult
> > ➤ Proportion based on child's weight.
> > > ➤ i.e., 125 mg bid for 35 lb, 250 mg bid 70 lb., etc.

or

Zovirax/Acyclovir
> ➤ 20 mg/kg/dose qid—5x/day (better)

Antifungals

It has always been a very difficult position to address clinically the possible role of fungi in the pathophysiology of any disease state, much less the symptoms of autistic dysfunction/NIDS seen in these children. Clinically, one presently looks for medical or lab support via low NK cell activity, elevated viral titers (as markers of a stressed immune system), and other markers for a stressed system (newer markers should make this justification much easier). Sometimes clinically one may see thrush, unexplained dermatitis, or ongoing fatigue.

Therapeutically, if a fungal overgrowth is present (in which case we assume a stressed GI system, propensity to yeast or fungal overgrowth, *not* the likelihood of systemic infection), this can be supported by the die-off or kill-off reaction. It is open to debate whether this represents a medical Jarisch-Herxheimer ("Herxheimer reaction") or a release of potential toxins (aldehydes) with lysis of the yeast/fungi. There is a period of more fatigue, more tiredness, usually more "spaciness"; then within usually ten to fourteen days the patient should be doing better clinically (sharper, brighter, healthier). If the die-off or kill-off lasts longer, one must suspect a problem or the possible need to change the antifungal. If there is a possible resistance, we must evaluate by medical decision whether improvement is occurring, the child needs some additional help or support, or it is better to proceed with changing the antifungal. Another issue of an ongoing negative reaction (usually different than straight die-off/kill-off) may be due to a medication formulation often not agreeing with that patient versus the straight medication itself. This is a potential issue with *any* medication used, particularly generics. These effects may be minimized by having pure compounds made, avoiding red dyes or liquids. (When using a liquid, try to stay grape or orange with the flavoring.)

While *Candida albicans* is arguably the single most important fungal pathogen, it is also a commensal organism, present in virtually all human beings from birth. It is ideally positioned to take immediate advantage of any weakness or debility in the host, and probably has few equals in the variety and severity of the infections for which it is responsible.[1] While we will research and fight for many years re the role of candida in different disease states, many of those issues are clearer if thought of as an opportunistic overgrowth, *not* as the primary cause of many symptoms or disorders it is often associated with. Clinically, there is abundant inferential evidence that both mucocutaneous and systemic candidiasis are typically associated with defects or weaknesses in the cell-mediated immune response.[2] They may reflect specific deficiencies in this context, such as in chronic vaginal candidiasis[3, 4] or chronic mucocutaneous candidiasis.[5] (One should note that while one might anticipate neurocognitive dysfunction in these states, it is not a primary focus of discussions. Significantly, these states do not account for or induce an "autistic" state of CNS dysfunction, seeming to help negate many metabolic theories that abnormal fungal metabolic products, seen in exceptionally high volume in these types of patients, induce "autism"—again support against yeast as the primary pathogen in many diseases with which it is supposedly associated!)

Epidemiological studies of *C. albicans* have been hampered by the lack of precise and reproducible methods for identifying isolates. Whatever the ultimate role and pathogenesis of candida, there seems to be no doubt that it can play a role in many pathologic conditions. As noted, yeast is certainly a potential pathogen in any immune dysfunction/dysregulated state. Yeast may be seen as a secondary phenomenon due to a generalized immune dysfunctional state (often documented by altered delayed hypersensitivity when tested). Clinically, it is not inconceivable that a yeast overgrowth in the GI tract can in theory interfere with nutrient absorption, altering amino acid and protein metabolism, thereby altering multiple body functions. I do believe that it is logical, if you are in an immune-dysregulatory state, you may be prone to an overgrowth in the GI tract. It is likely candida may play a role in what is referred to as the "leaky-gut" phenomena. Some physicians believe you have a toxin (an aldehyde derivative) released by the yeast and absorbed into the body, affecting the nervous system. Many physicians make the mistake of giving medication to control the yeast for only a few weeks or even a month and then stopping. If the patient was starting with a normal or healthy immune system this would be a very logical step. But working on the premise that a major part of the problem is the ongoing issue of the immune system dysfunction, trying to help it return to a healthy state, until it is there, and not offering some form of useful support is clinically foolish. In fact, one can argue that on-and-off therapy may be more inducive to resistance than some ongoing rotation of a maintenance therapy. (Again, with better true markers, we should be able to investigate this appropriately.) If, with treatment, a child becomes fully "normal," and their immune system is healthy, it is possible to withdraw all treatment and the child should remain healthy. Ultimately, the key is the body's own ability to keep appropriately in check an organism that it doesn't want to have there to start with. We are supposed to do that when we're healthy, but the body may have a problem when the immune system is stressed or compromised. At present, there is very little benefit to blood, stool, or urine testing for yeast or fungi. In a reputable lab, when any of these tests are positive, they are likely significant, but just because they are negative does not mean there is not a problem. (Note: Some of the children will have eosinophilia secondary to a parasite. One should not hesitate to send stool for O&P to a reputable lab if indicated.) All drug therapy is based on monitoring clinical and laboratory parameters with drug or dose modification as indicated.

Application

History of multiple ear and sinus infections with multiple antibiotics

Thrush or "suspicious" dermatitis along with markers of low NK cells raise significantly the likelihood of a fungal or yeast overgrowth in a child or adult

The idea of yeast or fungal overgrowth will be received skeptically until better markers facilitate accurate identification, but is interesting (particularly in children) how the symptoms seem to relate to yeast by-products (i.e., fermentation, drunkenness). If one thinks of altered delayed hypersensitivity as a component of the stressed immune systems, low NK cell function, the rationale, the idea of yeast as a superinfection becomes logical, just like we now recognize its potential role in many other immune related disorders.

Understanding the immune system, the concept of stress, opens the door to a rational discussion of the potential role of an antifungal in some of these children. With the high-level researchers I have worked with, if I said these children were the way they are because of yeast or candida, they would never have spoken to me again. I would have been foolish beyond that if I implied yeast or bacteria were loose in their bloodstream. If that was the case, adults or children like that would not only be in an intensive care unit, they would likely be dead. If instead I carefully came from the direction that we know from working with adults with this disorder that they frequently have what is called altered delayed hypersensitivity, then one can attempt to be rational, logical. We are taught as physicians that when delayed hypersensitivity is not working correctly, that is the part of our immune systems that is supposed to control and contain yeast and fungi—so when approached from that direction, there is justification to talk about applying an antifungal during a more controlled trial. It is critical to understand that if there is a likelihood of a yeast or fungal component in a child or adult with this disorder, it is because of the immune system being in a stressed state, not because it's a primary infection. I'll stress again, in light of the large amount of misinformation given to parents and adults, that if these children (or an adult) had evidence of yeast and fungi in their bloodstream, they would be critically ill in a hospital, not walking around with this mistaken label "autism." As discussed above with antivirals, if there's a real problem, real indication to use an antifungal, one must monitor its use (particularly the liver functions) and treat adequately. Consistent with infectious disease teaching, if one wants success, one must achieve a true remission, not go on and off antifungal choices at random, increasing the chance of making them ineffective, again creating more resistance. Once again, it is important to stress that when yeast or candida is present, it is a secondary, not a primary, pathogen, what we in medicine refer to as an opportunistic infection/pathogen. An antifungal if effective should cause what is called a "die-off," which will last from ten to fourteen days. A child or adult should use Advil, Motrin, or Tylenol for symptoms. If the child is improving, one may let the die-off go a little while longer. If it continues, it may be a chemical problem (with that agent) or resistance; either way you will have to switch to another medication. In theory, the healthier the child's body becomes, the less the need for a strong antifungal. Rather than starting or stopping at different intervals, it is a better principle to rotate antifungals every six to twelve months as long as they are needed.

CBC and chemistry panel are mandatory every one to two months.

There is no perfect test for candida. History is as important as any current test in making judgments for antifungal use

A trial with an antifungal (for now, until we have new markers available) may remain the best test for efficacy.

It is important that the parents check in during die-off, to be sure what is occurring is indeed die-off and not a reaction to the medication. The die-off usually lasts about seven to fourteen days, and after that time the change in the child can be rather dramatic. If the die-off does not end within fourteen to seventeen days, it is generally a reason to change choice of antifungal. (It may be an issue of resistance to medication or just a chemical reaction to that medication, particularly if it's a generic.)

If the treatment is being successful, usually eye contact improves. The children seem more tuned in and less "foggy." Parents will report that the frequency of inappropriate noises, teeth grinding, biting, hitting, hyperness, and aggressive behavior decreases. The children no longer act almost drunk by being silly and laughing inappropriately.

Sample Antifungals treatments:
(Initiate at ½ dosing for six days, then full)

Nizoral
- ➢ —4—5 mg/kg hs—max. 200 mg
  - • Generally change after six to eight months maximum.

- May have additional "immune" effect via "mild effect adrenal-cortical axis"—recent literature seems to support some direct effect on "neuroimmune" axis.

or

Diflucan
- ➤ —4—5 mg/kg hs—max 200 mg
  - Can be used longer term (per studies in other indications)
    - Limit to 1 yr. (before rotating)

or

Lamisil
- ➤ 250 mg (preferred for change over for maintenance rather than initial)
  - ~ 1/4 tablet 30—50 lb.
  - ~ 1/3 tablet 50—70 lb.
  - ~ 1/2 tablet 70—95 lb
  - ~ 3/4 tablet 95—120 lb
  - Full tablet above 120 lb.

The Potential Role (Limited) for Antibiotics

With the recognition of autism as a disease, a stressed and compromised but not broken immune system, opens the door, as discussed, to ideas of opportunistic organisms such as candida, and perhaps secondary chronic bacterial issues such as part of what we now call pediatric PANDAs. This was the recognition that somehow in the body, the presence of a chronic strep infection could trigger OCD (obsessive-compulsive) behaviors.[5, 6, 7, 8,]

Rather than long-term penicillin (not likely to be healthy for the GI tract), I use erythromycins usually. While sometimes an issue with GI tracts—stomachs (particularly in pill form, particularly in adults), I learned many years ago that while no longer considered a primary agent of choice, they were not only still effective (decades ago almost no resistance, now there is some), but unlike stronger antibiotics they were called bacteriostatic (they essentially paralyzed an organism, the body had to finish killing it off) rather than bacteriocidal (kill the organism directly). Because the body does not rush to kill off the "good guys," it was recognized many years ago (particularly with adults with CFS/CFIDS) that erythrocins and erythromycins (if tolerated) were least likely to disrupt the normal flora.

First working with CFS/CFIDS and missed ADHD in children and adolescents, many patients would present with what was being called a "red crescent" (inflammation of the oral—pharynx opening) and many had glands in the neck enlarged. Particularly when the anterior cervical glands (glands in the front of the neck) are enlarged, it raises suspicion of an infection. Since this infection is low grade, often chronic, one would not expect a routine throat culture to show much. Without a controlled university study, it was not appropriate to do "needle biopsies" for direct cultures (which would have to be extensive in searching for what might really be there) of what was there, leaving the option of ignoring these findings in an ill patient, or "compromise" and use a relatively nonoffensive, noncrucial agent (the erythrocins/erythromycins) to try to suppress or eradicate the infection. Not only was this very successful over the years (leaving open the ongoing issue that this, like so many other findings in these children, should be investigated, questioned, not just ignored or "written off"), but also it was my repeated observation (hard to call a child "placebo") that on an erythromycin/ erythrocin medication the child or adolescent would go to school, function successful, but off the erythromycin/erythrocin (similar names, different forms of same basic medicine: an old-fashioned antibiotic) would be bedridden or severely fatigued again.

It has been my experience that many parents would never have turned to alternative answers if the pediatric profession took an active role in diagnosing and treating these illnesses rather than taking a wait-and-see approach. I hope it is time pediatricians returned to being the primary doctors for "special needs" children, not observers from the sideline.

It is worth noting that if I were to be challenged with the question of what I was treating, I could reply I was not sure, but it was helping, and I was not creating likely harm. If I had advocated using a medication like Vancomycin, for example, without hard infectious disease evidence, that would have been irresponsible. To risk creating resistance to one of last major antibiotics used in hospital in life-threatening situations would have been negligent medicine. I stress again, that while a medication like erythromycin could be questioned, I have never, will not use stronger options unless they are directly indicated. It turns out, that with the information that erythromycins affect the "neuroimmune" system, one comes back to the question as to whether the medication is treating a bacterial infection or is it merely helping the neuroimmune system; for now my response remains "I don't care, as long as it is helping." To leave a child's brain and body fighting a disease they cannot win by themselves, to not support them with potentially safe agents, safe pharmaceutically clean agents, is not an option for me.

The place for SSRIs and limited other neurotropic agents

After diet elimination (always), antiviral use (usually), and antifungal use (frequently), then I will begin to consider the use of an SSRI. What is an SSRI? SSRI stands for serotonin selective reuptake inhibitor. What does that mean? When I was growing up, our parents often turned to prescription pills, then to medications like Librium and Valium as antidepressants. I can say from experience with NeuroSPECT, there would nothing beneficial about giving Librium or Valium to these children or their brains. While they have their place therapeutically, they are not going to make an adult or child's brain healthier. They essentially work by sedating areas that are involved in emotions such as depression in the brain.

The goal is to maximize a child's cognitive development. Therefore, the last goal to me as a pediatrician is to try to sedate or control a child. I would never choose to use SSRIs or recommend SSRIs as antidepressants. Unlike old-fashioned antidepressants that sedated the brain, essentially SSRIs do one job: they block the reuptake of serotonin being produced naturally and make it stay around longer. In this case, and fortuitously, the temporal lobes are primarily serotonin mediated. Since the key to this process is the neuroimmune-mediated shutdown of function, blood flow to critical areas of the temporal lobes, if I can take and block the reuptake of the serotonin being produced naturally (although they were not invented for this purpose), it's as close as I can come to titrate that area of the brain to get what one should be looking for therapeutically: first, a child or adult that wakes up rested in the morning, as if they had a good night's sleep and a healthy stage IV REM sleep cycle, and, second, a child (or adult) who looks bright, feels alert, as one would expect with any other healthy child.

In pediatrics we are taught to tell parents not to compare children, but in this case, it is true that your child should have a bright look to his or her face, as does any other healthy child. They may still be behind developomentally (takes time to catch up), but they must be there physically to succeed in the long run.

With the goal of long-term safety, I have stayed with what are called the simple SSRIs. Up to this point that means Prozac, Paxil, Zoloft, or Celexa. I avoid and do not believe in what are called complex SSRIs. It is very important to monitor a child for that sharpness, that alertness I have been writing about, and make sure that clinically you are not really inducing any negative side effects. While SSRIs can induce all sorts of reactions (which is the reason to introduce them carefully, slowly, with other variables controlled), they are physically very safe. Within negative side effects, one is looking for "zoniness," irritability, hyperness, or any response that, after time to adjust, is not in a positive direction for a healthier, better functioning brain/child. You are not asking an SSRI to control a virus, to control diet, or to control the immune system; rather, it is being asked to do one very important job, and this is help improve function in an area that has been sadly underworking, underused for a few years to many years.

While parents have been encouraged to by wary of SSRIs, and I do not myself concur with how they are used routinely, physical safety is generally not an issue. With SSRIs, while possible to throw a patient "off," with quoted risks including possible suicidal ideation, this is a mental issue (how does a medicine agree with someone, what "buttons" in the brain might it be pushing), but is not reflective of physical harm to the brain, a true physical toxicity. It is obvious that most of the side effects and most of the issues have come from these agents is how they agreed (or didn't) with any given individual patient. Even in the few reports suspicious of a true SSRI physical negative, the evidence is open to great debate, and may not sort out from what is called the background noise of patient selection and control of other variables.[9, 10, 11] Unfortunately, when listing side effects, the FDA does not make separate categories, and many agents, including aspirin, can look quite terrifying. It has certainly been my experience as a pediatrician, in using SSRIs for many years now, that until we analyze significantly more complex immune and biologic markers, or perhaps genetic markers, there is no simple way to choose what is the best individual SSRI for a child or adult.

Because the goal is to treat a physical dysfunction within the temporal lobes, if an SSRI did not agree with a patient, I did not give up on looking at an SSRI; I just had to adjust and make the right choices. Instead, in treating "depression," many psychiatrists might try an SSRI, but when that agent doesn't work, they move onto another class of antidepressant, and many are not looking to evaluate in any way the choice and dosing issues. It has been my experience that the choice of SSRI will change based on the brains state of development, not so much on a child's age, although in general, while physically safe, younger children may tend to get more hyper on Prozac.

Basing decisions on function, I am always looking to have a child wake up fully refreshed in the morning, having a healthy REM sleep cycle, and each adjustment of change must result progressively in a sharper, brighter child. Combined with other parts of The Goldberg Approach, the goal is ultimately to have a bright child, with a healthy sparkle in the eye, equivalent to any "healthy" child of comparable age. This is an extremely important concept to understand regarding the use of SSRIs and the whole approach to therapy being presented here. In my very early internship, after a few months of working in a very busy newborn nursery, while I learned to do screening exams, in reality I could look at a baby and know if that child was healthy or ill. There is a sparkle in the eyes a baby has, and, in theory, what a healthy child is supposed to have.

The choice of SSRI will likely change over the years. This will not be based on ideas of control of behavior, but it has been my strong experience that as the brain matures and become healthier, the best choice of SSRI will likely change. Very sadly, when you look at trials of medications for "autism," most trials are based on control of behaviors, control of aggression, control of "autism" symptoms. Even when anticonvulsants—which work by in essence decreasing nerve excitability thereby "dulling" the brain—may seem to have an initial positive effect for some of these children, dulling the CNS cannot in the long run be efficacious for any child. Since in the end we all need our brains working the best they can be, any medications that decrease function, slow down brain excitability, can only be a long-term negative. This is sadly confirmed that even for neurotypical children with epilepsy, anticonvulsants will ultimately lower IQs by a minimum of 5—10 percent (or more). Only SSRIs (in trials with "autistic" children) have shown to result in improvement in cognition and in a child's IQ and do not in theory carry a long-term physical risk (when used appropriately and judiciously). What caught my attention as I was dealing with chronic fatigue syndrome was that I heard about some adults who had been treated with Prozac, a new antidepressant medication. These adults were waking up rested in the morning. That meant that there was a considerable normalization of function that was occurring. It turns out that when the temporal lobes are underperfused, they are primarily serotonin mediated. Although it is not the whole answer to the problem, it was a tool that was not present with the earlier generation of antidepressants.

What I have learned in dealing with both adults and children is that if you can get them so that they are rested when they wake up, their brain is 98 percent where it ought to be.

Reasons for SSRI use:

> After combination of dietary elimination and appropriate symptomatic allergy control, antiviral (if indicated), and/or antifungal (if indicated).
  • *If* child is NOT fully bright and alert, *if* any residual spaciness, zoniness, or slow cognitive progress consider addition of SSRI.
> *If* hypoperfusion (particularly temporal lobe area) is present or remains on NeuroSPECT.

There is no absolute guideline or theory that says which SSRI will be the best for any given child. Always wait to start (with rare exceptions) until after child is stabilized on diet, antivirals and (if indicated) antifungals. SSRIs will increase blood flow to temporal lobes, by increasing function of those areas. They will have to be adjusted as the brain changes and matures (this has been a fascinating point clinically).

> Purpose/goal is to lift fog and zoniness and improve sleep cycles.
> If hyperness occurs and does not resolve in four to six days, change SSRI.

When one reviews medication trials for "autism," sadly the focus is calming behavior, controlling negatives, *not* improving cognition, ability to learn, etc. Utilizing NeuroSPECT, it may sadly be understood, that many of these medications being used to "calm" the brain and child down may further be shutting down function/flow in the very areas we need to improve.

What should be necessary to ask about every medical treatment or medication being used in these children is whether it results in a child who is brighter eyed, processes better, and functions quicker. In theory are you helping create a potentially healthier brain and child? Are there negatives associated with what has been prescribed? In theory, when treating a child, no negatives are acceptable.It can often be very hard to discriminate between what is behavioral and what is a medical issue. If you get a change where a child is more tuned in and processing better and in turn that child gives the parents or the teacher/therapist a "bad" time, this needs to be dealt with behaviorally, not medically. The time of adjustment, any changes physically (i.e., dietary, illness, allergies), must all be taken into account to sort out medication effects from behavioral or other factors going on.

I see in these children that the better their brain works, the more they initially act out like a two- or three-year-old kid who never had the "reins" put on them. If that's in the context of the brain working better, it's not a negative. One must be able to distinguish when a physically healthier, brighter child acts out at times from when a medication change is affecting a child physically or displaying itself in a negative mood or attitude.

It remains a complex process, like judging hyperness, anxiety, nervousness, and all these pieces simultaneously. I think these children are very anxious, I think they are very frustrated, I think they tend to act out a lot. I think they are miserable a lot of the time (*if* one speaks with older children or adults with similar disorders, their brains hurt them, their bodies hurt them—it has been my overwhelming experience they are not impervious to pain, they are just in a constant level of pain much of the time).

Often the more a medication calms anything down, the more it has the potential to shut off the areas you want to improve. Therefore, what you need to look at, what one really cares about with every medication adjustment or change is, is he or she brighter eyed, better processing, functioning quicker, physically healthier, or is there a negative? A major point with these children or adults is the simple concept of waking up refreshed, as a sign the brain is in a healthier place.

It has been my experience many times over to have a child doing better, processing better, but like any other kid, they'll have a bad day, they'll act out. If decisions are made on the basis of "we want a kid controlled and calm" (sadly still today, the "goal" of many therapists), you're never going to get the brain working right. However, if one makes a medication change, and you're getting a hyper kid, an irritable child, an ongoing negative, we don't want that change, and choices must be reevaluated. One must reconsider what the options are. But, if you get a change where the child, he or she is more tuned in, processing better, beginning to function as a "younger" child, and then causes problems (when he or she couldn't do so before), then that needs to be dealt with behaviorally (dealing with a child psychosocially, developmentally, age appropriately), *not* as "autism /PDD" and not as a medical problem.

A key point remains always interpreting where a child is psychosocially, developmentally, then dealing with that child, behaviorally, parentally as that child (for where they are developmentally—not their current chronological age), *not* the misconception of "autism/PDD—retardation." If a child is functioning bright and acting out, then you don't want to reinforce that, you don't won't to treat them like an infant and "redirect" or "refocus" them; instead you want to empower parents to act in a more normal manner.

When a child is being good, they deserve a response to positive reenforcements (important with any child). But *if* a child is misbehaving, a time-out (or for an older child withdrawal of a privilege or privileges) may be far more normal discipline for that parent and child. Sadly, part of the principles of any one discipline, is what does it cost that child, versus what they have gained. Children are bright enough to evaluate (as we do) what they lose (versus what they've gained). Any "behavioralist" giving advice to the parents of a child being treated appropriately has to understand the complete difference (again where is a child psychosocially, developmentally).

Here again is the issue of child recovering from a disease versus a behavioral or developmental disorder that in theory doesn't really change. As a physician, you need to constantly sort out and make the distinction: Is there a negative behavior because he's just acting out like a "typical" child, or is it negative behavior because you are throwing him off medically?

SSRIs—Neurotropics sample treatment
(always start low, work up at two- to three-week intervals
—or longer—toward optimal dosage)

Zoloft
- Large variability in dosing
- 5–10 mg/yr of age children

Paxil
- Approximately 1 mg/yr of age in children
- Do not exceed 40 mg in an adult

Celexa
- Generally seems to be about 2mg/yr of age
- Do not exceed 40 mg in an adult

Prozac
- Approximately 1mg/yr of age
- Do not exceed 40 mg in an adult

(Wellbutrin, Strattera, EffexorXR, or Tenex as indicated in specific cases)

Gamma Globulin Therapy

The idea of what is called gamma globulin therapy (IgG product) has been around for decades. At first there was significant risk warning about the IV form (IVGG), but that has thankfully become a very small (but still real) factor today. On the other hand, IM (intramuscular) use, while considered safer (extra step of acidification and processing), was not felt to be as efficacious (if at all) for serious disorders. Retrospectively the often "anecdotal" success of a "shot of gamma globulin" to boost someone's immune system while they traveled to Europe or a foreign country, which was done by a lot of clinicians, was never really proven in studies to be efficacious. As with any therapy application, too often, without an absolute guideline or marker, we are skeptical rather than inquisitive.

The debate regarding the efficiacy of gamma globulin, the ongoing fights regarding sugar and hyperness in children, and many other similar battles were all part of an early learning lesson—that what might be efficacious, and certainly accepted anecdotally as helpful or real, may not be easily or readily proven in formal, controlled studies. These were all clinical lessons, establishing for this author acceptance of the principal that there may be subpopulations for which a therapy may be significant, but not validated when looking at the whole / entire population. Especially when looking at these and other complex immune disorders, understanding, classifying the correct subpopulations is going to be critical to define successful therapies.

It is obvious over years of working with patients with this that some will benefit greatly (not just those with absolutely low IgG levels to begin with), but it was not going to be an answer for this disorder. In turn, expecting help, but not cure or resolution, unless absolutely indicated, I never wanted to use IVGG (even as the risk has thankfully become much smaller). Since IVGG is a pooled plasma product (as is IMGG), even with improved screening and virus neutralization procedures, the IVIG product carries some risk of transmitting viruses (particularly a retrovirus) and other biological agents.

It is well documented that experiences during infants' and toddlers' first months and years of life have a major impact on the evolving formation of neural connections, the laying down of "tracks" in developing brains. We develop brains over time.

When there has been a disruption in this process, such as the neuroimmune shutdown discussed in this book, it is not only important to help the correct areas of the brain—to open up, restore function—but then we must help re-create learning, developmental points missed in those early years. With brain functioning, the more this is done in a natural manner, helping a child not only learn but also experience or generalize something is a key to going back and "filling in the holes." We take it for granted, but these learning experiences lay the groundwork for that child to move on to higher learning, areas of comprehension, and so forth.

Back to the basic research, with the general acceptance that "experience shapes the developing structure of the brain" and the knowledge that the human body, including the brain, is made up of cells, it is only logical to start from a point that initially those cells may be somewhat organized, but they are nowhere near the level of function, the level of interconnections and "tracks" that will be need to function effectively as that child matures to become an adult. The idea that we cannot expect to reestablish or redevelop those connections is the ongoing mistake of the autism diagnosis and treatment. The fact that the brain is now known to develop into adulthood is a key reason for some optimism, even in older children.

Studies in brain physiology confirm that brain cells were perfectly designed for making connections. The cells signal each other; these electrical impulses travel down the cell and then are completed cell to cell by special chemicals (such as serotonin). It is the repeated activation and use of these tracks that ultimately results in a "mature" educated brain.

> Yes, there is a reason for homework. It helps to develop these brain tracks.

We must begin thinking of these children as potentially healthy productive teenagers, and adults. That means that we have to work to help them have a healthy potentially recoverable brain, not come from an assumption that somehow mysteriously that brain is predamaged, cannot be expected to function in a normal manner. I wonder how many of us would have succeeded if parts of our brain were shut down. Think of how many of the current "mixed" or "quiet" ADHD children are going to school as "space cadets." I feel extremely sorry for the teachers being asked to try and educate these children. Lack of recognition of the medical origin and severity of their condition may be a factor in what is looked upon as the "dumbing down" of our society. Maybe the common ideas of video games, parenting, teaching, and diet are factors, but what if they are not really the major ones at all? No wonder things do not seem to be getting any better for parents or children.

When approaching therapy, you must only change one variable in a patient at a time if you are going to have any controlled way of judging what the agent/therapy is doing. As I have expressed to parents many times, I would not have the general optimism, the literal expectation of a high level of success, if I did not go step by step. This principle seems to be forgotten with these children.

As much as I understand this disorder and have had physiologic insight (the NeuroSPECT) to the brain's actual dysfunction, I would not have had a chance to understand the many variables of a child if I did not go step by step. These principles do not seem to apply to most therapists recommending agents or advising parents on these children. Without following this approach, it is safe to say any therapist will find it impossible to sort out what is a physical change or a positive effect on the brain, from behavioral and other multiple variables in a potentially "normal" child.

When a three- or four-year-old, or a seven- or eight-year-old child starts acting out with the "terrible twos," one must critically be able to sort out good behavioral changes, likely normal developmental points, from dysfunctional or bad ones. As a pediatrician, as a person, as a parent, contrary to background or training, it became obvious in the early months of working with these children that they were children. How could a supposedly miswired, damaged brain pick up not where that child might be in chronological age, but developmentally, for many children, they would pick up back at that eighteen-month, two-year-old level, where they had in reality shut down (not been born developmentally or genetically miswired by some mysterious process). Some children of course were higher in function or abilities, but if not achieved in a normal way, were likely to have significant holes in their education or development.

I realized as a pediatrician to base educational and behavioral goals for the parents and the child, based on where they were developmentally (low points), not chronologically. As really applies to all of us, we do much better when all parts of our brain are working in balance, not underactive, not overactive. Using the NeuroSPECT, blood markers, and physiologic functioning helps guide choices or changes in therapy. Starting or stopping therapy/therapies without any attempt at objective markers, in my years of experience, is a very large mistake.

> I might have a child doing very well clinically, but the NeuroSPECT can still show that I still have not restored full function to the temporal lobes.

We need to raise our expectations of these children and understand this is a serious disease, not a developmental disability or a built-in genetic defect. What often may seem good enough under the guise of "autism," "ADHD," or other "LD" is not really nearly good enough if one starts thinking they began with a normal, or above-normal child.

If one understands we are not really looking at mysterious defective children (in a way too this day is not documented or validated by any objective markers within those labels, groups of symptoms), then one has to begin to seriously look at advice we give as pediatricians to parents about their children. Pediatricians and the medical world must step up to help parents of children do a better job in understanding them, parenting them, and dealing actively with their illness. They must realistically have a true goal of helping them to become more productive children, young adults, eventually independent, productive people (not forever dependent on social welfare). Working with this, particularly the severe-end autism, has been very eye-opening.

I often try to explain to parents that if you think of these children as children, it changes the entire approach to therapy; in reality we should all come back to basic pediatric training as an approach valid for any child that has been ill, not developmentally delayed or damaged in some mysterious manner. Once you get past medication choices, the restrictions of avoiding medications or supplements or therapy approaches (i.e., chelation, HBOT, etc.) that can harm a potentially normal child or brain, the next step becomes what everybody should be focusing on, which is how do you help to educate, to redevelop a child.

I can remember one of my early patients, a child who could not speak, but typed everything out on computer, and was obviously a very intelligent child. In fact, he eventually was in fourth grade in New York, attending and working in regular classes, but could not say a word. One day he was particularly misbehaving in his class, causing a very difficult time for the teacher and the school. Since I was due to see him for a consult in a few days, I asked the mother to have him explain why this was happening. I will never forget his note, a major learning experience. Essentially he wrote he was tired of being thought of as stupid, tired of people thinking he was dumb. He wanted a chance to learn more. How many behavioralists would remotely understand or give advice based on a child like this? If only others could understand the magnitude of what this child was feeling, so many others must be feeling. His mom and I were able to explain to him that we understood him, that if we were going to give him a chance to be in better classes, he had to be good in behavior, he could not get aggressive, he could not act out (even if frustrated with himself). From that day forward we were able to move the child into better classes, he became an excellent student, and eventually was able to be in regular classes in spite of the very difficult progress with language.

Referring to the child above who was in New York and not able to talk at nearly twelve years old, after moving to Washington, not classified under the autistic "label" any longer, he began to be able to talk, after receiving services from therapists who "would not take *no* for an answer!"

It's interesting to note that many of these children frequently have a heat or cold intolerance. Heat intolerance is a classic problem for many with autoimmune disorders—women with lupus often experience flare-ups on a hot or humid day. The lupus symptoms are often severely exaggerated under such conditions. I have an entire subgroup of children that show an outright heat intolerance, some mild, some severe.

As a child's brain and body become clearer, stronger, and healthier and it becomes possible to restore fine and gross motor areas, it is time to address the issues of apraxia affecting oral motor and speech.

I have seen many children go from awkward, resisting sport participation (even when brains were clearer), resisting writing (fine motor issues), to succeeding readily as member of sport teams, individually within their family (able to play ball with father, brother, or sister), and more. How many children do we allow to suffer when their brains and bodies are failing them, but are not broken, not really defective (in some mysterious way).

It has been my experience to see many older children and teenagers talk who had never talked before. This occurs with a combination of medical therapy, The Goldberg Approach, and excellent rehabilitative work by speech pathologists who understood oral motor apraxia, and were open to recognizing the medical nature of these children's dysfunction.

To not expect to be able to help a child get their language skills back under the guise of autism is not only doing a grave disservice to these children, but in reality, if you really think of them as children, you could begin to rationally argue that we are abusing these children. Very few "experts" that I have spoken with even remotely seem to understand how real the frustration is for these potentially above average to very intelligent children. In fact, understanding that many, likely most, of these children are starting off with above-average, sometimes brilliant potential, begins to change how one should be looking at, interpreting what we have called an "idiot savant." This concept has been that of an individual who is somehow expected to be retarded or below average in significant areas of function and ability because of their having "autism," while seeming brilliant (by accident, a mystery) in others. In reality, we need to begin to understand if the brilliant or above-average areas are that child's true ability. High functioning or "Asperger's" with its ongoing dysfunction is not really an acceptable end point. But these children are not approached with the concept of figuring out how to make the low areas healthy, how to really bring up, restore those functions.

The direction and the expected goals and needs of therapy must change. If one recognizes that they are working with a potentially normal or above normal child, one would never think of a repetitive manner of education as appropriate or even mentally healthy. If we think of ourselves as children, when a teacher asked us to write our names or something else on the board ten to twenty times, it was not to educate us, it was to punish us! If a child is being good and cooperating, they do not deserve to be punished. In fairness, *if* a child is completely zoney, completely spaced out, a benign, modified ABA type of approach may be justified (better than nothing), but if a child is brightening up, and his or her brain is beginning to work, therapy goals and approach must change with that child.

It remains my strong belief that if we begin to look at these children the right way—as sufferers of a disease—many capable pediatric developmental specialists, good child psychiatrists, and well-trained therapists will know how to help those children far better than the ideas being currently being used or proposed. The ideal of rehabilitating a child carries over even stronger when it comes to speech. I learned early that to try to teach a child, have them say what might be a stage III or stage IV skill, before stage I or II have been developed, is a mistake. This makes sense physiologically, as we are taught as physicians and therapists, that when the brain learns developmental/functional steps out of order, it is often harder to undo that and harder to correct that. To achieve fluency, a chance for normal function, one must always work from the bottom up. This applies to speech and to all areas of child development.

If we go back to reality, back to the fact these children are ill children, then speech therapists almost automatically will go back to their basic training. As pediatricians and speech pathologists, we are trained in school that when any child has delays early in life, multiple ear infections, any serious illness or dysfunction altering their normal development, their development of language, you need to restart from the earliest skills. You didn't step in and just try to get words from that child; instead you had to go back and help redevelop their early skills. Speech professionals are taught to start with six-month skills, then eight-month, ten-month, one-year skills, working their way up the developmental ladder. Without a full background, how many "neurotypical" children could talk correctly? How does a child under the label of "autism" have a chance, when we do not approach them with any of the effort and expectations we apply to a potentially normal child? Working with an excellent speech pathologist oriented toward rehabilitation (think of your children as a stroke victim rather than a child with autism), it was my early pleasure to see ten-, twelve-, fourteen-year-olds begin to talk, when they could not talk before. Sadly, it has been my ongoing frustration with children who are becoming very bright and alert that they often do not receive the proper therapy tools to have the potential to recover language the way they should.

One of my first patients with this was a child from fairly wealthy parents in Philadelphia. Over a two-year period we documented return of normal function in his temporal lobes; clinically he was appearing as a bright and alert child, and yet in spite of working with the "best speech therapists in Philadelphia", he could not say one word. Beginning to learn about and understand this, I told them he needed a speech pathologist who understood rehabilitation. Being very motivated, these parents found a "rehab speech pathologist." First evaluation session with the child, the rehab pathologist tells the parents, "Your child cannot talk, he cannot even stick out his tongue!" The "top people" this child had been seeing for two years had never approached this child as they would have any "neurotypical" child who had delays.

Focusing on using therapy to obtain a bright, alert, healthy child, many updates and follow-up discussions circle back to how I trained, what I was accustomed to as a general pediatrician. How do you help a parent deal with a child behaviorally, and most important, how do you try to optimize a healthy child developmentally? This background has turned out to be a major area helping me with these children. As stated earlier, you must have the expertise to evaluate a child, based on where they are developmentally, which should in turn guide behavioral, educational, and developmental needs. If it's a seven-year-old child who is only a two-year-old developmentally, you must parent, discipline, praise, educate, and work with that child as a two-year-old, not the seven-year chronological age. If it's a fifteen-year-old, and he's a five- or seven-year-old, you must deal with that child appropriately. As I have found with minor adjustments and understanding of background frustrations, difficulties, you parent a child very much as you would a normal two-year-old, five-year-old, or seven-year-old. These children are frequently redirected and refocused instead of given appropriate consequence or behavioral corrections for a child functioning at their age range. No normal child grows up without a mixture of love and discipline. Treating these children like they cannot understand correction often makes them much worse behaviorally and educationally.

The success of many of these higher expectations—the right to parent a child as a potentially normal child with delays—depends upon a child being bright, being alert, being able to process. So I will partly qualify that you cannot expect these results until you've also looked at the medical side of therapy, but if you have been looking to medical therapy and a child is brighter and functioning better, then one must think and respond appropriately as a parent, as a pediatrician. It is perhaps wiser to try to work with a child, even if he or she is still zoney, assuming they are intelligent, rather than allow bad habits to develop (which are then harder to undo).

As a a pediatrician, you might tell a parent of a six-month-old, one-year-old, and even perhaps when an eighteen-month-old child is reaching for something on the table, going or doing something appropriately, you in essence might redirect them, refocus them. But somewhere by two, two and a half, if that child doesn't respond to caution and parental guidance, they do not listen to the parent, most parents are then going to begin to institute some type of time-out, some type of consequence. It has been my very sad experience to realize that we make many of these children into disasters behaviorally, not because they have to be, but because we don't discipline or help them in the way we would a normal child.

Is it is very hard to expect a normal child to grow up okay, without a mixture of love and discipline. All love is usually not good, all discipline is usually not good. So again, it is a situation that if you think of these children as likely damaged, retarded, unfortunately you might think of redirecting, refocusing them, using only positive reinforcements. But if you think of them as an ill, but potentially normal or above-normal child, as noted, behavioral and education advice and goals change dramatically.

Also, I must stress that clearing a child medically, helping them be able to feel better, is critical from a number of directions, including the fact that how much of what is thought of as behavioral acting-out or self-injury is really because these children are miserable, they are in pain (headaches, body aches), not just because they are choosing to be difficult or misbehave. Help relieve that discomfort, help clear up the brain, help a child be able to begin to comprehend, and then you can work with that child in a much more positive, healthier, more normal method and pattern.

> I was advised how many of these children seemed to be impervious to pain. Just the opposite has been my experience. Help them return to normal functioning physiologically, and they feel pain just like any other child. However, when in constant pain, constant discomfort, what's a little more at times?

I have said to many parents over the years that *if* experts really understood what was happening to these children, we would be calling it child abuse *if* we thought of these children as anything but "autistic." While we are more civilized, PC, use the term "special needs," the implication remains an expected level of retardation, instead of a normal or significantly above normal IQ.

As noted, the NeuroSPECT has helped me tremendously over the years, first to begin to define and understand this dysfunction, and then to be able to guide me with ongoing clinical management and therapies. While many clinical decisions become obvious over time, instead of assumptions or educated ideas, the NeuroSPECT is like a road map, showing what is working or not working in the brain.

After the initial steps above, after usually initiating an SSRI (interactions in the temporal lobe directly influence the frontal lobes and other areas of the brain), I will then attempt to focus on what is left residually abnormal in the brain. If a child is doing well, but there is still temporal lobe hypoperfusion, it is going to be a reason to reevaluate each step of therapy, and if indicated, potentially change choice of SSRI. If there is what is called frontal lobe hyperperfusion (increased blood flow), after controlling diet, eliminating supplements and any other products that might be irritating the GI tract or stimulating the brain or both, I will consider agents such as Wellbutrin or Strattera. Both seem to affect the norepinephrine-dopanergic system, potentially helping to regulate these areas, in what again *if* used judiciously, used to restore physiologic functioning, seems to be very safe long-term.

It turns out an old-fashioned medication called Tenex has a significant place in children, adolescents, and young adults with this dysfunction. While it was originally classified as a blood pressure medication, as a pediatrician I was introduced to it as a medication for children who were hyper, but too young for stimulant meds (which I have never believed in, and have a very limited constructive application). Now, while it can be used for hyperness in a younger child (with hyperfrontality—to some degree physiologic in some children), it has been extremely constructive in addressing basal ganglia, deeper brain stem hyperperfusion. As it turns out, Dr. Ismael Mena was able to validate that this hyperperfusion was due to inflammation; therefore I have come to look at compensating for that as another positive step in balancing the brain. If hyperperfusion is present on NeuroSPECT, I will use Tenex, never to sedate a child or adult, but rather to help improve function, overall sharpness, and alertness.

A special-ed teacher, who started with me as a teenager with ADHD and fatigue, on a recent scan had some basal ganglia hyperperfusion (increased blood flow in deeper areas of the brain). She started on low-dose Tenex, and while not complaining previously, on follow-up she commented she could settle down, fall asleep easier, her brain could get into gear and stay on task easier.

Why are we not applying new technologies, using new abilities to make more educated, directed judgments in any attempt to diagnose a learning dysfunction in a child and with any application of a neurotropic agent. How much harm do physicians allow to happen iatrogenically, by not using newer imaging, new tools in a far more constructive manner? Happily, the NeuroSPECT has helped guide therapy decisions for me while continuing to push for access to agents, therapies that could in theory end this one day for children and adults.

I am opposed to any neurotropic agent that does not act in a manner one can rationalize as healthy for the patient or their brain. Most meds acting in a neurotropic manner would never meet this criterion. Sadly, among the many medications being given more and more frequently to children (and adults) are what are called stimulant medications. The starting point was Ritalin and old-fashioned amphetamines, but most newer ones are merely variations of the same. Sadly, parents are not told that any of these stimulant-based medications are just like giving a child cocaine. There are many studies in the literature now supporting that Ritalin is just like cocaine, only stronger. I've yet to see a study saying or implying a brain was healthier with cocaine. While sometimes, with the general stresses these children's brain have been through, I have been encouraged to be open to *very low* dosages; I remain quite concerned that at normal dosing, especially when used with a mixed or quiet ADHD child, particularly with no SSRI support of the temporal lobes, one has a high chance of decreasing function in key, critical cognitive areas of their brains. Sadly, as noted previously, this misuse may now be a key reason contributing to the ongoing discussions of the "dumbing-down" of our school-age children.

When working with a child (or adult), one must start with a reminder that like any person, any biological organism, these children have multiple variables that may affect their moods, their actions, their attitudes, their performance. Not understanding these are potentially normal children who are uncomfortable, do not feel good, is missing part of the immediate battle to do the right thing to help that child (or adult). It is a completely different tactic or response when a child is acting out because they do not feel well, are in pain, versus the oppositional behavior or attempts to resist learning of a child who is now brighter and in theory does feel much better, but just doesn't want to cooperate. Just like any of us, these children become much more receptive to learning, much more productive, when their brains are functioning, not foggy or zoney, not constantly uncomfortable. I would politely challenge any reader of this book how they would have done in school (educationally or developmentally) if in a constant fog or zone, often in pain. In no other area is the crossover more graphic than thinking about the spaciness, zoneyness, brain-fog of a child with autism/PDD, a child with the new, now majority mixed or quiet ADHD, most adults now labeled ADHD, and an adolescent or adult with what has continued to be called facetiously chronic fatigue syndrome/CFIDS.

As noted, understanding this first through the eyes of adults and teenagers suffering from the early days of "complex neuroimmune, complex viral illness" has helped me as a pediatrician and as a person to understand these frequently nonverbal children. Older children and adults would often describe their headaches as "the brain felt like it was going in twenty thousand directions at one time." They have a whole syndrome, fibromyalgia (essentially this disorder in adults with more physical then "mental" dysfunctions) describing multiple trigger points, tenderness, and areas of pain. As noted previously, most therapists and physicians dealing with these children do not think of this, do not have any more insight into the true nature of disorder, than the experts from the CDC who first coined the name "yuppie flu" to put down and label psychosomatic this disorder in previously high-functioning adults. I frequently wonder if we might have ended this disaster medically before it grew larger if we had approached those adults with an open mind, if we had understood something was physiologically wrong and had studied it, tried to figure out objectively what really was going on. The psychiatric implications first condemned the adults, and now so many children, to be misdiagnosed and misunderstood at a critical time for them and for our society. Without bringing about a true recognition, and the urgency for research and real answers, health, education, and welfare costs can only continue to spiral out of control until the system collapses!

Combine all the mistakes about this disorder, the failure to recognize both its sufferers' cognitive potential and likewise the amount of pain, dysfunction, and discomfort they are in, and we are torturing these children and their families. Years ago, beginning to realize how completely distorted, broken, the "system" had become, I began to say quite cautiously to parents that "heaven forbid," but they would be better off dealing with a child with cancer than with "autism." A few years ago, I met a father who had a child who had autism and another who had cancer, and he was openly telling other parents it was easier to deal with the child with cancer than with the child with autism. It is my sincere hope that if the crisis comes back to the medical world, where it belongs in the first place, we would change this and approach it for the children and their families just like cancer, just like TB, just like other infectious diseases, in this case much more chronic.

Falsely believing in a mysterious developmental disorder, we have not approached these children and their problems with the urgency they deserve. This deserves the magnitude, and more, of any effort for polio, measles, cancer, and any other critical childhood illness. We must create a pediatric, medical, and social world that helps support these children and their families, and recognizes that as science is supporting, that if it is not predamaged, the brain has a tremendous potential for recovery and redevelopment. As noted above, if we understand we are not born with mature bodies or brains, but must use and develop them, then the understanding of how to help redevelop a child is already out there for all of you—we just need to recognize and deal with the real problem.

8

MISTAKES AND MISDIRECTIONS

Mercury

OVER THE YEARS MANY MISTAKES HAVE been made, and continue to be made, in trying to explain the mysterious causes for the outbreak of autism and other cognitive dysfunction in children and adults. For me, any idea not based on logic or science has never had a chance of providing answers. Yet, after first convincing adults why they now have CFS/CFIDS or adult ADHD due to heavy metals, toxins, multiple different environmental or other metabolic arguments, the same logic, the same therapies are being sold to these frantic parents and their sadly dysfunctional but ill children. Like what happened in adults, unless they address primary causes, the primary reasons for dysfunction, a lot of efforts may seem to help a child for a short time, but they are not going to continue to help or likely be even safe longer term, and this is supported by a mounting number of long-term failures. Accepting these limits and these problems are part of the mistake in thinking these disorders are somehow developmental and can't be helped otherwise.

For instance, we are taught in medical school that lead and other heavy metals are not good for the brain. The key is, as pediatricians we were never taught that there was any connection between heavy metals and autism. To make up or imagine "undetectable" levels of heavy metals, particularly when those heavy metals cannot cause "autistic" symptoms, cannot and will never explain this growing epidemic of ill children.

With mercury poisoning, the characteristic motor findings are ataxia, dysarthria, and spasticity. In autism, the only common motor manifestations are repetitive behaviors (stereotypies) such as flapping, circling, or rocking.

As part of this dysfunction, there has been a dramatic increase in children on the spectrum with fine and sometimes gross motor issues, children with levels of hypotonia. To me, none of this is compatible with old ideas of autism, and there is nothing in multiple peer-reviewed medical literature articles to support this type of motor changes arising from mercury or other heavy metals. If a child did present with ataxia and/or dysarthria, along with autistic behaviors, then a careful medical evaluation, looking for an alternative or additional factor, is justified.

While a characteristic sensory finding of mercury poisoning is a highly specific bilateral constriction of visual fields, not only has this not been reported in children on the spectrum, but the sensory defensiveness of autism is more likely related to altered sensory processing within the brain itself, rather than a peripheral nerve involvement more typically seen with metal poisoning.

Other signs that may appear in children with chronic mercury toxicity, such as hypertension, skin eruption, and thrombocytopenia, are seldom seen in autism. When mercury poisoning occurs in prenatal life or early infancy, head size tends to be small, and microcephaly is common. Microcephaly is not common with ASD, and there are literature publications supporting general macrocephaly (larger brains) or enlargement of particular parts of the brain in children with autism. It's worth noting that in typical exposures to neurotoxins, the tendency becomes, again, decreased head size. In spite of the obvious differences noted above, in spite of the fact that after more than fifteen years of study, in spite of the fact no paper published in the peer-reviewed literature has supported or reported an abnormal body burden of mercury, or an excess of mercury in hair, urine, or blood, how many parents are asked to do chelation for their children to clear their body of toxic (often not measurable) toxins/metals? Parents are not told that these children do not have signs of true mercury or metal toxicity and that they fail to have detectable levels by any standardized, accepted lab testing technique. Nor are parents told the fact that in multiple pediatric studies, in multiple pediatric lectures, we are taught to be concerned about the potential for harm from chelation itself. (Note: Supported strongly by recent FDA reports on the dangers of chelator agents). With recent finding that DMSA (a common chleating agent) is toxic to mouse and rat brains, no prescription medication I would prescribe for a child now or in the future will ever have that level of toxicity. When I graduated from medical school, you were taught that you would chelate a child with a lead level of 15 to 20. Now, current teaching is to think of chelation at 60 or 70, and to chelate above 70 or 80. Why did this recommendation change? Not because lead is good or less toxic, but because in controlled studies, something yet to be done by any group advocating chelation for children with autism, it was found by the American Academy of Pediatrics that in cases of lead poisoning, except at higher levels, children who were chelated often did worse than children who were not. When one understands how metabolically off these children are (secondary to the immune system, low NK cells, abnormal mitochondrial function—not built-in defects), one can understand the number of anecdotal reports of children seeming to be helped by chelation. By now the lack of long-term gains or changes should make many more parents suspicious, and the complete failure of any published report to support chelation confirms that the likelihood of long-term harm, probably highly exceeds any real chance of gain or success. Consider that with the known toxicity of DMSA (and likely other chelating agents) and the negative potentials of chelation itself, when applied to a presumable autistic child, how many children have been hurt without it being documented or verifiable? This should be terrifying to readers of this book and many other organizations or societies dedicated to protecting children and helping parents. When did we enter a society where frantic, desperate parents are allowed to be led down false and potentially harmful paths for treating their children, while the real medical world, the pediatric world I trained with and grew up respecting, stands by letting it happen, partly innocently, and by now at least partly inexcusably.

Sadly, talking about misleading information, while parents were presented with multiple arguments how barely detectable mercury had somehow done this to their children, in real life, in the real world there were studies looking at contamininated seafood in Japan and Iraq (and reports from health departments in multiple countries in the world, particularly those that consumed a lot of fish) showing the effects of mercury toxicity, and none showed an association with autism or autistic symptoms. In fact, on autopsy reports, there were significant decrease of neurons, increase of glial cells, macrophages, a short frontal lobe, and lack of definition of the cortical layers. Not only are none of these findings characteristic of children with autism, but, in fact, a finding of atrophy of the cerebellar granule cell layer with relative sparing of Purkinje cells is in direct contradiction to new and old reports on brains of children with autism, showing loss of Purkinje cells, not sparing of those cells. It's time to stop chasing impossible stories and ideas and bring together a hard focus, a call for true science, logic now, or as many have now seen, this will continue on the path it is, benefiting some, but destroying many.

Multiple studies in credible, peer-reviewed journals followed victims of high-dose acute or chronic mercury poisoning resulting from contaminated foods in Iraq, Pakistan, Guatemala, and Ghana. Again, none has reported manifestations suggestive of autism in survivors. In contrast, many of these survivors had clinical signs such as persisting ataxia and dysarthria that are seldom seen in autism. In autopsies of people with autism one finds no reports of significant cerebral cortical neuronal loss or calcarine atrophy. Frequently, autistic forebrains unusually show small, closely packed neurons and increased cell-packing density. Portions of the limbic system are consistent with curtailment of development of this circuitry. (Note: Curtailment of development is consistent with a neuroimmune shutdown of blood flow and function, *not* being born mysteriously defective to begin with.) As noted, another consistent finding in the neuropathology of autism is reduction in Purkinje cells in the cerebellum, primarily in the posterior inferior hemispheres.

Involvement of granule cells has rarely been reported, while in contrast, mercury-exposed brains have shown significant and consistent damage to the cerebellar granule cell layer with relative preservation of Purkinje cells as previously noted.

Finally, but also ignored by all those who so strongly advocated mercury (or heavy metals) as a cause of autism, in our history, during the first half of the twentieth century, mercury was a common constituent of medications. Use of those mercury-containing compounds was associated with illness in young children, typically those between eight months and two years old, reflecting typical symptoms of photophobia, anorexia, skin eruption, and bright pink color of hands and feet. This was called "pink disease" or acrodynia. Survivors were not described to have behavioral disorders suggestive of autism.

Issues of mercury poisoning go back many years in Japan, including epidemics of methyl mercury poisoning back in the 1950s in Manamata and the 1960s in Niigata. Heavy prenatal exposure resulted in low birth weight, microcephaly, profound developmental delay, cerebral palsy, deafness, blindness, and seizures. Affected adults experienced impairments of speech, constriction of visual fields, ataxia, sensory disturbance, and tremor. Was autism recognized with higher frequency in Japanese children in the period of these toxic outbreaks? Japanese reports in the English language do not indicate that Japanese clinicians thought so!

In summary: While mercury poisoning and autism both affect the central nervous system, specific sites of involvement in brain and the brain cell types affected are different in the two disorders as evidenced clinically and by neuropathology. Overall the clinical picture of mercurism throughout history doesn't mimic that of autism.

It's again worth noting that most of the ideas claiming mercury or heavy metals in children with autism were also similarly proposed first to explain adults with the strange disorder of CFS/CFIDS. In these "proposed" disease models (MS, CFS/CFIDS, fibromyalgia) exposures such as maternal Hg exposures (e.g., from vaccinations, thimerosal-containing RhoGam injections during pregnancy, or dental fillings) have been ruled out repeatedly in the literature as having no connection to causation or reason.

Vaccines

Very sadly, also contributing to lack of focus on the real medical crisis is the failure to bring to the forefront the real medical world and the pharmaceutical industry (yes, your children need them as allies). In addition to blaming metals, the linkage of thimerosal to vaccines became a great case for physicians and clinicians who have long been opposed to vaccines, to now have a large audience of desperate parents willing to listen and unfortunately believe.

When one looks at the concept of combined stresses on the immune system, particularly stresses of possibly multiple vaccines in a sick, not fully healthy child, the chance that vaccines may be one of the combination of stresses leading to that autoimmune point is very real. The temporal relationship may at times let them seem to be possible "triggers," but they are not the cause of this disorder/epidemic. The misdirection of parent anger and frustration at this point has only served to slow up real progress for these children.

Since I trained as a pediatrician with a good background in immunology and infectious disease, I was more than aware of childhood illnesses like measles, mumps, chicken pox, polio, and more. The fact is that the real diseases, the natural diseases, both mild and severe, were not associated ever (except fetal exposure to maternal rubella) with causation or cases of autism. This is supported by the fact that during decades where there were childhood epidemics of these disorders, the rate of something called autism was so rare (1–2/10,000) that as late as the 1970s, I and other pediatricians were still being told that if we saw one "autistic" child in the lifetime of our pediatric practice, it would be one too many. Needless to say, with many practices having six to twelve such patients now, that rule is long gone. To want to focus on and blame vaccines for the change now has never been and will never be good scientific reasoning or logic. By now it should be criminal to mislead so many innocent families (and their children) who do not have a medical education or background to understand the many fallacies of the ideas being presented. During early days of basic science in the first year of medical school, we spent a significant amount of time learning how to dissect a medical (or other) article. As physicians we spend years of medical training to try to learn how to sort out logic from science fiction, possibilities from reality. Asking parents to do that when they have no medical background is reprehensible.

I want to to stress again, there is a wealth of data supporting the lack of causation. Understanding the role of vaccination as a potential "trigger" and helping to remove their potential role as immune stressors in any child is important. As a pediatrician, I have followed a policy of supporting necessary, important vaccinations for every child, including many high-risk families, without ever having a vaccination lead to any kind of a lasting problem. Consistent with my medical school training, my pediatric internship and residency experience, I have never given a vaccine in the nursery (the most dangerous time in a child's early life), I do not give six or eight vaccines at one time (but if a child is fully well, that might be okay), and I never give a vaccine to a child who is ill. It has been my experience that if I explain to a mother her child is ill, and ask her to please bring him or her back when well, the mothers in my practice have been likely to do so (or we might have a strong discussion by their next exam). Because some parents won't come back, because some might be unreliable, was it ever a good policy to give so many vaccines to so many ill children? These are issues that should be studied further, looked at, and understood in terms of immune stress, not just classical ideas looked at under the concept of "vaccine injuries." The ideas of NIDS presented in this book are not defending or looking at the role of vaccines in regard to causing or creating "autism." That will never be the case; it's time to move on.

Some feel autism has never been described as a mercury-induced disease simply because the disorder must arise from a mode of mercury administration that has not been studied before. In fact, mercury (Hg)—its symptoms, methods of detection, negative effects, etc.—has been studied for many, many years. There is no support for the link between mercury in vaccines and autism in past literature.[1]

In 1999, family physicians, pediatricians, federal health officials, and vaccine manufacturers stated that because any potential risk from mercury is of concern, and the elimination of exposure to mercury in the form of thimerosal from vaccines is feasible, thimerosal should be removed from vaccines as soon as possible. However, there remains no convincing evidence of harm caused by low levels of thimerosal in vaccines.

This theory does not account for the children who have never had any vaccinations or "heavy metal" exposure.

NOTE: *If* vaccines were connected, between the decrease in thimeresol and decreased vaccine "exposure" (the number of children not being vaccinated), there would have been some decrease (not current increase) in California (much less other parts of the country and the world). High metal levels are not being found by academy-accepted accredited laboratories (university-level children's hospitals).

Chelation Therapy

Skeptics have consistently criticized the lack of adequate controls in studies purporting to demonstrate the effectiveness of chelation. Critics of the therapy in the American Medical Association (AMA) and the Federal Drug Administration (FDA) claim that there is no good scientific evidence supporting the extravagant claims of advocates. Defenders of the therapy claim that the medical establishment has engaged in a half century of deceit and conspiracy to suppress chelation because of fear it would cut into the profits made by drug therapy and surgery.

Most human chelators are a form of protein containing thiols, also called sulfhydryls, meaning a sulfur and hydrogen compound. Sulfa drugs are known to be deadly for people who are intolerant. ("Autistic" individuals are noted to have sulfur issues.) Most of the drug versions are synthetic molecules, molecules created by man and not naturally found in humans. There is the possibility of the body's not being able to metabolize such compounds, resulting in allergic reactions, autoimmune reactions, redistribution of mercury, and other dysfunctions. The bottom line will be your body's ability to expel the chelating agent along with accumulated mercury. If your liver and kidneys are not able to push out the chelator, you have a problem. If your body cannot excrete the chelating agent, it will need to metabolize the material, breaking it down to its constituent parts. The mercury gathered by the chelator will be dispersed into your body again, rapidly, as a large dose. Such a rapid redistribution can magnify your mercury toxicity problems.

CNS toxicity (of chelation): Dr. Haley, PhD, has shown that EDTA can cause release of mercury in a form a hundred times more toxic to the brain. Severe damage to the brain tubulins can occur, resulting in Alzheimer's-like dementia.

Hair Analysis

The AMA's Current Policy on *Hair Analysis*—Adopted in 1984 and Reaffirmed in 1994 is, "The AMA opposes chemical analysis of the hair as a determinant of the need for medical therapy and supports informing the American public and appropriate governmental agencies of this unproven practice and its potential for health care fraud." (Hair analysis: A potential for medical abuse. Policy number H 175. 995, Sub. Res. 67, I-84; Reaffirmed by CLRPD Rep. 3—I-94).

In 1999, researchers from the California Department of Health located nine laboratories and sent identical samples to six of them. The reported mineral levels, the alleged significance of the findings, and the recommendations made in the reports differed widely from one to another. The researchers concluded that the procedure is still unreliable and recommended that government agencies act vigorously to protect consumers (Hair analysis: A potential for medical abuse. Policy number H-175.995, Sub. Res. 67, I-84; Reaffirmed by CLRPD Rep. 3—I-94).

Even if hair mineral content were measurable with 100 percent accuracy, it makes no difference because the results are not useful for measuring the body's nutritional status.

Should you encounter a practitioner who claims otherwise, run for the nearest exit!

DMSA

DMSA is approved for the treatment of lead poisoning, and it can also remove essential minerals such as calcium and iron. Thus DMSA has potentially serious side effects for developing children.

To put things in perspective, a trial funded by the U.S. National Institute of Mental Health (NIMH) was halted because an October 2006 online study in *Environmental Health Perspectives* examined the impact of DMSA on rodents, showing direct neurotoxicity from the DMSA. Because of potential dangers to test subjects (120 autistic children aged four to ten) as implied by the studies on rodents, the proposed "experiment" was canceled (see why below), along with the recognition that it never should have been proposed in the first place.

A lot of research is being done that proposes to counter false ideas, false concepts, rather than focus, as the case should be, on finding answers. In this way the "multiple misdirections" proposed and being done are not just benign, but rather have slowed down coming to a constructive, correct focus for parents and their children.

In the experiment, after undergoing three weeks of chelation therapy with oral DMSA, what surprised the researchers was that animals that were not lead poisoned showed "lasting emotional and cognitive problems" after undergoing chelation therapy with DMSA. The researchers did not know the reason for this. However, they speculated that DMSA might have caused the non–lead poisoned rats to lose essential nutritional minerals since there was no lead to bind to the drug.

There are two other chelation compounds commonly known as EDTA: disodium EDTA and calcium disodium EDTA; the former can be dangerous because it removes calcium from the blood.

Given the Academy of Pediatrics' recognized position against the risks and dangers of chelation, even for indications of known toxins such as lead, no parent should allow a child to undergo chelation without a university or children's medical center documenting the need.

In a recent conversation with a lady and her husband supposedly "in the know" I was told there were now "thirty-seven kinds of autism." Not forty, not twenty-five, but thirty-seven. This is the most illogical, ridiculous rationale I can ever believe could circulate. We do not have thirty-seven (or any other number) forms of autism. We maybe have one form that Dr. Kanner described, and then multiple variations (twenty, forty, thirty-seven, or more) of a "complex immune, complex viral" illness that one can now talk about as NIDS, and explain logically, with good science and medical reasoning, not via the "myth of autism."

While as physicians we are taught to think of an illness as mild, moderate, or severe, autism and related psychiatric disorders were not defined or thought of that way.

What has happened to common sense?

A list not necessarily in order of treatments that are common in the autism community:

- Purine metabolism
- Phenol metabolism
- ABA
- Anticonvulsants—EEGs
- Steroids
- Megavitamins
- LDN (low dose naltrexone)
- Secretin
- Enzymes
- Probiotics
- Special diets
- Chelation therapy
- Hyperbaric oxygen therapy
- Stem cell therapy
- Electroconvulsive therapy

- Religious interventions
- Educational interventions
- Sensory integration
- Vitamin B6 and magnesium
- Vitamin A—cod liver oil
- Essential fatty acids
- Casein-free diet
- Gluten-free diet
- Cognitive/Behavioral therapy
- DMG
- Melatonin
- Homeopathy
- Auditory integration training
- Ritalin (or other stimulant medication)
- Risperdal or Abilify
- Seroquel
- Pepcid
- Buspar
- Intravenous immunoglobulin
- Inderal
- Play therapy
- Vision therapy
- Sound therapies
- Neurofeedback

Besides outright toxicity from "natural" agents, I learned an agent being extensively recommended to help with sleep, melatonin, was in fact probably worse than a prescription sleeping medication (something I would not recommend), as melatonin had the potential to play with multiple hormones in boys (some in girls). That means it is not safe to use regularly, and if used at all, should be treated like a sleeping pill, perhaps used once or twice a week, never on a regular basis.

As noted before, not only are these agents usually not specific, but with most not being pharmaceutically clean, there is more chance of creating harm, than of helping (even if a theoretically good product to begin with).

As noted, many "natural" agents are quite toxic, and especially with children, anything megadosed is not going to be safe. Replacing a deficit (if real) can be appropriate, but overdoing that usually will result in harm. Again, the key is first a recognition a child is ill, but being ill means the medical world, pediatricians, and other pediatric specialists can and must look at applying agents to help a child (or adult) win a medical battle they have been losing, but not by using agents that are likely to result in harm. If we recognize a child is not "damaged" mysteriously to begin with, agents that have high potential to damage the development of a normal brain (i.e., antipsychotics) become unacceptable.

I cannot stress strongly enough that supportive, appropriate use of medications has never resulted in the potential harmful effects currently being seen on NeuroSPECTs of children who have been doing supplements, chelation, HBOT, and such.

I have been saying for years that you can probably do one hundred or more things that might seem to help these children, in lieu of how dysfunctional their bodies are metabolically, but unless you're doing something that you can sustain in a healthy way, a healthy manner for that child, it is rare to see initial gains continue, and more than likely harm may occur over time.

If we raise expectations, recognize this is a disease, and bring these children back to pediatrics, then expectations will rise, and parents have a right to expect that we will truly "do no harm."

I am still working with a patient that first came over from England, not as an infant, but as an eighteen-year-old. He had completed high school with accommodations, essentially working at about a third- or fourth-grade level. But because he grew up in England, and although academics were not helping or supportive, this was an era when what is called the "DAN protocol" or "biomedical" was not commonly accepted, and so this mother had never administered megadosages of vitamins or supplements, chelation, HBOT, etc. The mother did try to watch his diet, but that was essentially all she did. This child's response to therapy at age eighteen was easier for me than children I was seeing here in the United States who unfortunately had undergone massive supplements, chelation, hyperbaric oxygen, and other related "therapies." This has been confirmed by NeuroSPECT scans showing not only were the areas of dysfunction not being corrected but areas always previously normal on scans were now under- or, more often, overstimulated, which was confirmed by NeuroSPECT scan.

Recently, I have begun to give mothers and fathers a guarantee that their child can not really have "autism," as the term is being used today. Recently, as noted, numbers of affected children in this country are routinely being quoted as 1:110, or 1:91. Main theories still remain focused on a mysterious genetic/developmental disorder, but it is now safe to say that in the history of written medicine, back to at least the middle ages, there is no record of any developmental/genetic disorder remotely coming close to a 1 percent number. When parents ask what really *does* strike 1 percent or more of a population, my response is, a massive flu epidemic, the bubonic plague, STDs, maybe. The point is, anything affecting 1 percent of a population is going to be a serious disease or medical illness.

When a mother is empowered and believes her child has the possibility to be healthy, she can begin to respond far more appropriately, as she normally would, to a child that is being good, a child that is misbehaving, a child that is happy, a child that doesn't feel good. I remind mothers that while they didn't plan on all of this when they were younger, they will, unlike many parents, be able to look back and know they had a chance to really help their child have a productive and ultimately healthy life—what more can any parent (or doctor) ask for? It would just be nice to make the battle easier, simpler, but either way they have a right to be proud of themselves for choosing a fight that is difficult but that can be won. For not accepting many educated voices saying they must accept and must give in to "reality." For not seeking pathways in desperation that might be harmful. Ironically, the first lesson in pediatrics at medical school at UCLA was "listen to the mothers."

How often does this emotional turmoil and dysfunction create family conflicts in the attempt to care for these children? How often do families wind up splitting apart, making attempts at unified care even harder if not impossible? Again the key comes to how mothers and father are asked to perceive their child. It's hard to live in a world where multiple experts will support that if this happens to your child, you can do your best, but it is unlikely you are ever going to have a normal parenthood or a normal child. We owe parents the truth, the knowledge that *yes this is bad, yes this could be very difficult*, but as parents, they can fight against a disease that their child has a chance to win. Mothers and fathers come in to my practice ecstatic after they hear their child first say "I love you" or they put their shoes on for the first time. Why shouldn't parents have the right to know they have a right to expect that from their child? Especially when there is *no objective evidence showing or confirming permanent damage to their child's brain*!

The understanding of the true nature of this illness has certainly helped hold many families together—and thankfully even when it's a belated recognition, can help separated parents work together on their child. Like a child with diabetes there is a need for proper diet control. Like a child with cancer, a chronic viral illness, or an autoimmune disease, there is a need for supportive medication and an ongoing need to maintain therapy.

Just like any other disease, I believe it should become negligent not to take part, support the medical care of a child, whether parents are together or separated. Like a child with any other serious illness, the standardization of therapy and the diagnosis is critically necessary to assure expected consistency from household to household for a child.

9

THE ROLE OF ALLERGENS AND DIET

LONG AGO I INCORPORATED DIET ELIMINATION as part of my pediatric practice. In particular, I would often caution against the use of dairy products. While common sense and good clinicians were aware that dairy (the number 1 allergen in the world) could lead to or add to congestion, this was not "proven" and was contrary to the conventional wisdom at the time. Fortunately, my training at LAC-USC included the teachings of an allergist who strongly believed in food elimination. But I did have parents leaving the practice because other doctors were telling them that there was nothing wrong with dairy products and they felt I was misguided. I had also been influenced very heavily by Dr. Frank Oski, a leading pediatric hematologist, who later became chief of pediatrics at Johns Hopkins Hospital. He was lecturing that dairy products could cause iron deficiency in children and that could then impact their growth and development.

Today, there is plenty of information in the medical literature about the dangers of dairy products and of milk protein. But we still do not have the technology to know of all possible forms of allergic reactions to milk or dairy products. My disillusionment with modern medicine stems from the concept that if it cannot be measured, it must be a psychiatric problem or not real—rather than an acknowledgment that we do not have the tools to measure the problem.

I usually begin with blood testing to determine allergies/sensitivities that could possibly trigger the immune system to react. Most children with autism/NIDS (and all of its labels) present with routine sensitivities to dairy, whole grains, nuts, tropical fruits, and often berries. While often confirmed on testing, these are common allergens in any child or adult with an overly reactive immune system. We deal with local environmental factors as indicated (allergens like pollen, grass, pollution). As noted under prevention, I remain a strong proponent of judicious use of inhalers to both block reactions and control inflammation. Frequently these children will appear allergic to a large number of foods, not necessarily because they are allergic to everything being tested, but rather because their immune systems are so dysfunctional, so overactive, that they react to almost everything. This reaction may or may not occur as asthma, a rash, or hives. It's clear now that *all* negative foods, impurities in many nonpharmaceutical grade supplements, sometimes even different fillers in generic medications, can contribute to or accentuate this immune mediated, abnormal "shutdown" of blood flow in the brain that affects the language and social skills areas of the brain and central nervous system function. While accentuating the negative shutdown (think of a rise and fall in alertness, zoniness in a child—often day to day, sometimes hour to hour), as noted it is now known and well studied in the pediatric epileptic literature that immune activation can directly lead to a greater propensity for seizures (the immune system attacks, and therefore activates, foci in the brain).

By just placing the patient on a diet free from dairy products, chocolate, and whole wheat, one can see an immediate improvement in function caused presumably by a lessening of immune system stress, reducing inflammation of the brain. Again, the presumed reason for this is to help by removing a trigger, reducing stress on the immune system. This has nothing to do with the false idea of GF/CF (removes dairy and gluten but then adds "other" whole-grain products with their own negatives), but with the now recognized fact that while "bovine protein" is the number one allergen in the world, wheat and other grains is number two. If dairy, milk chocolate, and whole wheat are taken away, as much as 98 percent of probable allergies are alleviated. However, while often a very helpful start, and critically important over time, I do not believe that you can correct this condition by diet alone. If this were possible, parents (and physicians) by now would have heard of multiple, "unbelievable" successes over the years. Reputable institutions would be conducting clinical trials to investigate the successes. Since nutritional therapies have not resulted in cures, or even published reports of significantly improved cognitive function, it is illogical, in fact potentially detrimental, to put these children on extreme diets. However, sometimes these children put themselves on extreme diets by only eating a limited number of foods. I don't think there are a lot of normal children who would be healthy on some of the diets these children put themselves on. Since these children are often drawn to and even crave negatives like a drug addict, this is often a helpful clue to tell parents what to avoid (even if a child seems to go through a withdrawal, that will be far better long-term for that child).

For most of the children, all that is necessary is to eliminate the "main offenders" in their diets that will cause the immune system to react. It is not necessary to eliminate all wheat (but over time, restriction of grain-based carbs has become more and more important/critical). Some doctors and homeopaths recommend the elimination of all gluten and wheat. I feel strongly at this point that the reason so many of these children show initial (but not long-term) improvement when they are put on a gluten/wheat free diet is they no longer are eating whole wheat or have dairy! Usually, all that is really needed is to eliminate whole wheat and other whole grains (due to allergenic potential) from the diet, not the full extreme of GF/CF (but I do have a few children that seem to benefit from the extremely limited diet, even though they do not have celiac disease).

Many parents comment how after just the initial food/dietary phase that their children become more manageable and more amenable to reason. Some to the extreme of beginning to talk that did not talk before. One should not underestimate or ignore the potential reactivity of the immune system, and various foods, proteins, peptides, or other sensitivities (while these areas need better clinical markers and standards, till "proven" it is an area one cannot just ignore, but must approach with logic and reason). If a parent notices a good effect from a diet elimination, effort should be made to support the family in their search for other "logical" exclusions. Unless there is a very significant jump, "extremes" are usually not necessary or justified (particularly in children). What I have experienced clinically is that as a child begins to do better, it is easier to judge what throws him or her off. You need to be expecting a general continuous upswing (or consistency from medical agents); if there is variability, try to think what did he/she have to eat before a decline. What was done differently? One must stay very "tuned in" with the parents to pick out variables and problems. It is useful to keep a diary, particularly tracking "off" times, when there is no immediate, obvious answer.

I never cease to be amazed at how many parents will say "my child is allergic to milk," but then the kids are still getting cheese or other dairy products. The truth is, you don't see as bad a reaction to a processed product as you do to a healthier, natural product. This is part of the whole argument, when you get into nutrition, about processing something, how you change the protein structure. So a child that might go berserk on milk may not appear weird on processed cheese. But if a product is a negative, in this type of reactive system, any exposure is not good. The concept that when you change the protein structure, you frequently alter its allergenic characteristics was illustrated early in my pediatric practice. A child could do well on formula for twelve months, but when switched to milk, the introduction of dairy products, one will observe diarrhea or congestion, the start of chronic stuffiness, other signs of allergies (recurrent ear infections, sinusitis, etc.). A child may react to milk, but seem to tolerate the cheese. The trouble with the philosophy of "tolerance" or rotation is if you understand the reactive immune system, anything firing it off further is not helping. The child may not be over the edge when you see red ears or some other "tolerable" reaction, but you're still firing off that body and the immune system behind it. So it's really worth being very strict. Many parents, particularly early along, did not recognize how important a factor this is. Occasionally, rarely down the line, especially a child that was not real high on food screens with dairy or some food they particularly want, I'll say to go cheat (*very* hesitantly, *very* cautiously, almost never at this time). It gets very easy if a child's doing well, and they receive something "illegal" or forbidden. It will become obvious very quickly if you're throwing them off or not. If you're not, (and there is *no* evidence of increased eosinophilia on blood work) an occasional cheat may be okay. A sugar treat is better than a dairy or other such reactive treat as it leaves the body more rapidy then the effects of dairy, and does not activate the immune system. A dairy treat can throw the immune system off for seven to ten days or longer, so if your child cheats once a week, this can be a serious impediment to progress. A key common issue in therapy is separating when one is dealing with the normal issues of postnasal drip or other environmental allergies versus when a cold or allergy has turned into a sinus infection. Typically, the ideal of a "postnasal drip" is a child who has a little sniffle or is congested in the morning (upon waking), perhaps a minor cough or two, but is then generally clear the rest of the day, maybe becoming a little congested again by the evening. If that congestion is continuing most of the day, for more than a few days, odds are high the child is moving from just allergy, to at least a low-grade sinus infection, or early fluid in the ears. Likewise, if a child has external allergy exposure or food allergy (not good), they may become congested at times, but again, should be an off-and-on situation, unless constant exposure, constant error in diet choices leads to the emergence of a chronic sinus or ear condition. The crossing over from "just" allergies, to a cold, to sinus infection, is important to recognize and understand clinically, for any time these children are ill, any time they legitimately do not feel well, they are not going to do as well. A key role in removing stresses, helping a child (or adult) become healthier is prevention of illness whenever possible, and then treat, and assist the child judiciously in handling an infection, rather than allowing a major stress to set them back or weaken them further. In a heavy orientation to prevention, particularly in regard to allergies, I was fortunately taught to think of how to keep a child (or adult) clear, avoid repeated complications, rather than just treat recurrent complications and infections.

Long before antihistamines or decongestants were in common use, doctors were left to diagnose and treat each ear infection as it developed. By being preventative in my practice and treating congestion and mild fluid aggressively, I rarely had a child with a major infection requiring heavier antibiotics and have never had a child admitted to the hospital for more serious complications. In my many years of practice, I've had very few children require ear tubes.

Prevention is a key to keeping a child healthy by removing stress on his or her immune system. As discussed, diet is a key starting point always. But *if* a patient lives in an area surrounded by pollen (perhaps everywhere but the part of L.A. I live in) or spends the day in a classroom environment open to molds and other contaminants, then the use of "preventative" inhalers becomes a very safe and wise move. Nasalcrom or Astellin are for the nose and nasal passages, Intal or Tilade for the chest. These are key choices to help prevent inflammation, reactions, infections, but if a child is ill, congested, or fighting a sinus or chest infection, they in theory do not hurt, but really do nothing at that point to treat the infection (but may help in preventing ongoing stress, exposure during recovery).

Prevention carries over to the routine use of what are termed "nighttime" twelve- or twenty-four-hour antihistamines. The goal is to use a slow-release antihistamine that does not cause any clinical side effects (child does not awake tired or hyper), but helps that child start off the day clear. This idea of prevention is illustrated by how the simple step of avoiding chronic (overnight) inflammation to the throat prevents the lowering of resistance common when the mucosa of the throat is inflamed. What we call an intact mucosa is a key to helping a child (or adult) resist the many infectious agents they may come in contact with at school or elsewhere. By preserving an intact mucosa, the first barrier to protecting against entry by many respiratory, throat, and ear pathogens, one is going to have a child with a much better chance of staying healthy, in spite of their "allergy" tendencies. The use of an effective nighttime antihistamine and judicious choice of inhalers often ends the need for other antihistamines or systemic medications during the day.

With many of the children, it can become very deceptive when on surface they appear to be doing very well, but they do not yet a fully "normalized" immune system. By "well," I mean tuned in, cognitively connected, alert, processing on their own, learning quicker, doing the steps you expect the brain to be doing. I've received frequent "panic calls," the child's off the wall; they're doing this and doing that. Usually (particularly when no recent medication change) the child will be coming down sick or they've gotten strawberries, cherries, dairy, or something else to eat that day (throwing them off significantly).

The Dos and Do Nots of the Diet

As noted, many of these children have major allergies or intolerances to many chemicals and foods (understood in terms of activated immune system, immune sensitivities, and not always true allergies). The main offenders appear to be cow's milk, wheat (and potentially other whole grains), and salicylates (among multiple chemical sensitivities noted). Occasionally these reactions may turn into urticaria or asthma, but in the majority of these children the effect is the concept of activating, triggering a system one is trying to calm down. This often results in a worsening of autistic-like or negative behaviors, physically a zonier or often more irritable child. Interestingly, the family history of these children often reveals eczema, migraines (especially in mothers), hay fever, and asthma.

These children may often crave the very thing that does them harm (reflects the negative idea of a brain addicted to a drug, rather than the brain or body craving what it really needs). They do this not only with foods, but also nonfood items they ingest, mouth suck, or chew (e.g., metal, plastic, perfume, soap, plastic, dirt, etc.). Frequently, these children become picky eaters at the time they "change," eating only a few different foods and both craving some and avoiding some. Some autistic children begin to eat nonfood items with notable immoderation. It is important to encourage the child to eat more protein. This will help balance out naturally their own amino acids, which in turn is part of helping their bodies become healthier. All these children need protein. It is also necessary to restrict starches. Healthy breakfasts, lunches, and dinners should be served.

One should:

Avoid all dairy, chocolate, whole wheat, and whole grains—while limiting sugars. This does not mean to replace them with equally allergic grains easily available at heath food stores.

All dairy means any product that has milk or bovine protein listed as a "major" ingredient.

This includes cheese, yogurt, chips with cheese on them (Doritos, Cheetos, etc.).

Common sense and logic fall back onto basic principles taught through my training programs. Bovine protein is the number one allergen in the world. With the recognition that in somebody with a reactive, sensitive immune system, just like a virus particularly a flu bug can trigger off the immune system in any individual, so can bovine protein exposure in a reactive individual. Whether a virus, or bovine protein, the immune system makes a mistake, attacks the pancreas; and in some cases a person can becomes diabetic for the rest of their life. This happened to my wife. In this discussion lays an explanation for what many say is "most confusing" regarding the dietary advice I give. We have grown up with the concept that whole grains are what are good for us, and with a food pyramid that was saying we needed six portions of grain. As a physician it remains my experience that biology is what runs us, and we evolved primarily as carnivores (yes, we can eat other things, but our muscles and our brain builds on the basis of amino acids. Growth is extremely difficult to maintain in a child from just plant sources), so WHO decided we needed six portions of grains a day. If we were living two hundred or two thousand years ago, maybe the argument that whole grains were better than "processed" would hold up, make sense, but in this case, anything reactive (a major characteristic of whole grains) is going to do far more harm to the body than good. Perhaps we need to get back to the advice of the 1950s or 1960s—meat, vegetable, and some fruit, a little bit of carbohydrates. In that advice think of it as if your grandparents didn't eat it, maybe you shouldn't, either. How many products do you eat without additives and chemicals? We need to go back to eating food, not chemicals. Unfortunately, whole grains are the number two allergen in the world; this has created a terrible mistake in many children. The initial, mistaken concept these children might have something called celiac disease, produced the ideal of the gluten-free/casein-free diet recommendations. As noted, while some children may initially improve upon removal of dairy and gluten, when one takes away dairy and gluten but substitutes other whole grains, it has been my sad experience to see many children come in with a more reactive immune system, more reactive food screens being created by GF/CF. While counterintuitive, after years of being accused of borderline quackery to think of diet elimination, a university-based MD and PhD gave the mother of one of my patients even more reasons to be concerned about organic meats. While "organic" (no pesticides, etc.) might be a healthy way to grow an acceptable fruit or vegetable, this researcher (and his colleagues) are seeing a tremendous problem with organic meat. Instead of "organic" meaning grass-fed, or naturally fed, many of the cows are being fed whole grains, which are going through the meat to the children ingesting it. This has completely "muddied" the concept of natural, organic (particulary when it comes to meats). There are ranchers who will argue that all of this comes back to physiology—cows were not meant to eat corn (apparently it really changes their meat in other ways). For now, grass fed, naturally fed, whether labeled organic or not, is probably the safest step. Perhaps some of the milk and meat sensitivities would be nonexistent if cows were just fed grass (like years ago). Initially this whole issue would have been illogical to me, as the concept of processing, cooking, and heating changes many of the proteins. Many years ago I treated a child who was so sensitive that his allergy cells, eosinophils, would go up when given milk-fed veal! So contrary to the idea heat treating changed this, it has become obvious that these children (perhaps most of us) are much better off with range-fed, grass-fed, naturally-fed meat, rather than just trusting or buying "organic."

The reason for this is physiologic—if you start recognizing the correct problem, you can start to think correctly. Under the ideal of gluten-free/casein-free you are removing gluten but often using other grains, other whole grains as substitutes. Unfortunately these substitute grains to these children are just as reactive, if not more so, than gluten. In fact a few years back, a patient that had been with me for a while was doing well overall but had ongoing allergy issues, came back after the mother had dropped out of the practice for a while. She was an intelligent mom, did not fall into doing anything foolish or considered dangerous to her child, but did try gluten-free/casein-free. This child, who had a very high IgE while in the practice, an IgE of 700 (Note: in the mid-late 1980s, I sent a teenager to UCLA for an IgE of 700, never before having seen a number that high—now this number and higher ones have become routine), this child came back on a gluten-free/casein-free diet, with an IgE of greater than 2200! Since grains are considered allergenic, it is a wise idea to limit carbohydrates in these children. Ironically, many of these children are attracted to carbohydrates, leading to a crossover discussion that these children, perhaps like drug addicts, are wanting to consume something that is harmful to the brain and body. As noted, it is almost always fair for a mother to assume that if a child is craving something, loving something, be suspicious. Although a large amount of carbohydrates is not ideal, it is safer for these children to consume carbs derived from simple potato. For instance a potato chip may be much safer, if a child is old enough, than any gluten-free/casein-free pretzel. Perhaps the only real need for bread in these children should be a sandwich at lunchtime. In that circumstance, many times, well-processed, inexpensive white bread is less allergenic than any GFCF bread with other whole-grain substitutes. In the rare circumstance that the child does react to that white bread, then very carefully look for a choice that is not going to trigger allergies.

These children have extremely reactive GI tracts. I will always remove red cherries, strawberries, watermelon, and most berries to start with. Interestingly, it was originally a Dr. Feingold who proposed removing sugars and reds in children that were hyperactive many years ago. At that time I certainly agreed with removing sugars in children that were hyperactive, but over the years it has become obvious that he may also be right about the idea of red dyes. I would add even natural red. "Reds" seem to be something that can trigger many of these children along with blues (the reason for removing blueberries). Many physicians will dispute or continue to argue against anything we can't fully validate. Instead of being open to the possibility of a problem, if it can't be measured we assume it is not real, rather than an unexplained possibility. Interestingly, a few years ago, there was a news story about a woman who was violently allergic to strawberries; in fact, she would die if she ate a normal strawberry. However, she was able to eat a synthetic *white* strawberry. As a physician I only can dream or how far ahead we would be today if we had studied what we don't understand, what we don't know; instead of redoing what we've already validated or believe is likely to have a high probability of a successful, predicted outcome.

With these children (with rare exception, caution) it is very wise to remove nuts. Ironically nuts and citrus are number three and four in food allergies when we are taught about potential food sensitivities, potentially reactive food groups. With general certainty, these children will react to nuts. Among the many dietary mistakes is the idea that you take away dairy, but then should be substituting a nut-butter-based milk instead. This is almost as big a mistake as giving a child dairy. Unfortunately any natural nut milk is going to be potentially very reactive.

It is only with great caution and care that I will okay a child eating processed creamy peanut butter as part of a sandwich for lunch. First only with the recognition that we have to be able to give children something for lunch and the old standby "peanut butter and jelly" sandwiches may have to cautiously be a part of that. While children will often go off the wall on crunchy or natural "wholesome" nut butters, as with wheat, the processing that goes into making that processed creamy peanut butter helps to reduce the allergy potential in a child sensitive to peanuts.

Because of how sensitive these children are, there is an ongoing need to take time to isolate and control variables. A mother observing her child noted that one brand of processed creamy butter seemed to be fine, while on the other brand, the child would rapidly become hyper. The difference was that the "bad" brand had molasses in it. This leads into discussion again that any impurities are potential problems. The reason honey is often not good for these children (including the risk of botulism below twelve to eighteen months in any child) is that it's not a clean product.

So in general nuts, with the additional fact that they contain arginine that can feed these herpes viruses, should be avoided. There is an additional reason, perhaps interconnected to the sensitivity issues discussed. Nuts become "rancid," and they produce trace toxins which may impact beyond immune sensitivities. Depending upon the food screen, I do find some children should be removed from citrus. In addition to nuts, citrus is a surprisingly common source of food allergies.

I will always recommend a child be off reds and tropical foods (not native to the region). From that point it will depend on what else may be significant on a patient's food screen, but of course no test is perfect. Whether one does the newer blood-based RAST testing, which is IgE based, the old-fashioned skin testing that was IgE based, or the newer IgG4 screens, no testing is perfect and no parent should be told that because a child is negative on a test, that means that food is okay. As an example, we have known for years as physicians that IgE testing is fraught with problems such that if a child is positive in an IgE based test they are likely to be allergic, but if a child is negative they could still be allergic. With the IgG4 food screens many products may appear reactive, overly reactive, reflecting the overall activation of the immune system. So one must carefully look at and interpret patterns with logic. No child is likely to be allergic to everything being tested, but sometimes can be so overly reactive that everything appears to have what we call a marked "shift to the right." While not absolute, when a follow-up test shows cooled-down immune reactivity, many past offenders now become nonreactive and that is a good sign the immune system is becoming healthier and less stressed. This creates a very nice picture of what the child's immune system is really doing.

Don't deprive your child, however. Substitutes are always available for almost any product. Children seem to really enjoy "fake milk" in place of milk available at most health food stores and more and more markets depending on where you live. Easier to find are soy milks and sometimes goat's milk. But remember, there is about a 25 percent cross over between dairy and soy allergies, and the more natural, the more "organic" the soy (or even the goat's milk), the higher the chance of a sensitivity/reaction. It's a wise idea to get your milk pasteurized. Mocha mix nondairy milk substitute is available at most supermarkets, as well as mocha mix ice cream.

Fake cheeses are also readily available. TofuRella comes in cheddar, mozzarella, and jalapeno for the brave. These melt and make a reasonable fake pizza or fake grilled cheese sandwich. There are many other brands of soy cheeses—make sure there is no added milk protein in them. Goat's cheese is often a good choice (and tastes pretty good).

Chocolate is an offender, because most chocolate is "milk chocolate." An occasional treat made with cocoa powder or nondairy dark chocolate is usually feasible.

With any "new" food always watch for a reaction. If your child has a reaction, that product is not for them. Breakfast should generally consist of some "processed" (meaning not whole-grain) cereals such as "Rice Krispies," or Corn Flakes unsweetened, served with one of the fake milks. Some children have a problem with the preservatives put in cereal, especially BHT. If this is your child, then a preservative-free cereal like puffed white rice or rice squares will sometimes work (be cautious, always avoid products made from brown rice). The key issue with *any* grain is how well processed or "clean" it is (even white rice).

Again, a lot of these children also have problems with red, yellow, and blue food dyes. Pay attention to your child if they consume these in cereal or fake candy and watch for a reaction. A "diet" soda is a great reward as long as your child does not react to NutraSweet or Splenda. Sparkling flavored mineral water is a good choice with no added sweetener. Most sugarless candies can now be found sweetened with saccharin, Splenda, or NutraSweet. Sorbitol also works as a laxative so keep an eye out for loose stools.

In general, limit sugars.

The average American consumes more than 120 pounds of sugar a year. For example, a hamburger bun has three teaspoons of sugar; a regular nondiet twelve-ounce soda has nine teaspoons of sugar (regular Coke, 7-Up, Sprite, etc.).

Other names for sugar to watch out for on food labels:

- Brown sugar
- Corn syrup

- Dextrose
- Fructose
- "Natural" fruit juice
- Galactose
- Glucose
- Jam
- Jelly
- Lactose
- Maltose
- Maple syrup

Water down juices, start with half water/half juice and work down to one-fourth juice the rest water. Be creative. If your child loves those juice boxes, pour them out when the child is asleep, refill with diluted juice, and put a piece of scotch tape over the top. You'll get away with it. Kids love the new Crystal Light drinks that come in sport bottles. Buy them once, then refill the bottles with the Crystal Light you can mix at home. Or use the single packaged portions you just add to a bottle of water.

Lunch is a good time for leftovers and extra protein.

Protein supplies necessary amino acids, which are the building blocks of the body. No supplement can do as well as the real thing. Lunch is a hard meal to really make healthy. A sandwich is okay as long as some protein is in the middle. Bread is where the controversy begins. As long as your child is not overly gluten sensitive or has a significant titer to what is called gliadian antibodies, "processed" white bread is generally okay. The word wheat is okay as long as the word "whole" is not in front of it (but this can be very confusing). The reasoning is, many people are allergic/reactive to whole grains, but not as dramatically, if at all to a processed product. Processing, changing the protein structure, grain, etc., removes most of the allergenic properties. For this reason, often the store's cheapest white bread is a good choice because when it costs less, it is less likely to have butter and other allergenic ingredients in it. While this may sound horrible for nutrition, the idea is not for a child to eat a loaf of bread, but to use it as a way to sneak in the protein (as part of a sandwich). Be careful—many white breads advertise whole grains; these are not the ones to feed your child. Besides allergens, whole grains are much harder to digest and can increase intestinal inflammation. I am not arguing nutrition but a simple way (bread) to get the child to eat protein, have a sandwhich for lunch at school (not at other meals).

Dinner can be any meat, chicken, fish (if tolerated) with some vegetables and a little starch (small serving of potatos preferable, occasionally white rice, very white processed pasta). Try to remember the body converts starch to sugar within a few steps, so that is another reason to limit consumption. We know your child may be stubborn at first and only eat the starch on the plate. The key is not to argue with them—if they do not want to eat the rest of the food, do not force them. But do not let them fill up on junk food/more starches/sugar, "grazing" either. When they want more food, present what they have not finished or just say "wait till the next meal" (either approach is okay). Believe it or not, their pattern of eating will change. Too often parents give in and become afraid a child "will starve to death." The key is to understand that brain is often craving what is bad for it (like a drug), and in the end you are helping your child to control those cravings. As a pediatrician I can safely say "there are no reports in this country of a child starving to death, if offered food." Remember, you cannot make a child eat (or go to the bathroom), but "nature" will work for you if you let it. Getting a child healthier, and a judicious use of iron (when indicated) helps to stimulate, bring about a more natural appetite (which makes it easier to then modify or change things). Install a good water filter in your home if there is any issue of toxins or possible problems with your water supply.

What can my child eat?

- All meats (avoid milk-fed veal, organic beef fed with whole grains)
- Fish all kinds (not prebreaded)
- Seafood such as whitefish, salmon, shrimp/prawns
- Be cautious, sometimes increased allergy issues with shellfish
- Poultry such as chicken, Cornish hen, turkey

- Eggs (unless the child has eczema)
- Celery
- Cucumber
- Dill, basil, rosemary, thyme, oregano, etc.
- Fennel
- Lettuce, romaine, escarole, endive, radicchio, etc.
- Olives
- Radishes
- Red/green peppers (bell peppers)
- Artichoke hearts
- Asparagus
- Aubergine (eggplant)
- Avocado (use caution, can be a problem)
- Bamboo shoots
- Bean sprouts
- Beet greens
- Broccoli
- Brussels sprouts
- Cabbage
- Cauliflower
- Celeriac
- Chard
- Green/French beans
- Kale
- Kohlrabi
- Leeks
- Marrow
- Okra
- Pumpkin (be cautious, sometimes a problem)
- Rhubarb
- Spring onions (scallions)
- Spinach
- Summer squash

- Turnips
- Water chestnuts

Fruit

- Apples
- Apricots
- Bananas
- Cantaloupe (be cautious—may be a problem at times)
- Pears
- Grapes
- Peaches
- Plums
- Orange (if not a problem with citrus)
- Fruit juices—limited quantity. Water down to reduce natural sugar content (not fruit punch or red coloring)

10

○ ○ ○ ○ ◎ ○ ○ ○

TIPS TO HELP GET
THROUGH THE DAY
(DEPENDING ON BEHAVIORAL AGE)

B EHAVIOR: TREAT AS A NORMAL REGULAR child, adjusting for age developmentally. Time-out initially. Then as older developmentally, the child loses something for the day (something child really enjoys). Helps to have a behavior chart at school. Gets a smile (overall OK or good) or frown (bad day, aggressive behavior, etc.) from teacher end of the day. If child comes home with smile, great. If a frown, the child loses something major (i.e., all electronics) for the rest of the day. Start fresh the next day. (Note: No daily bribery, but like for any child, if a week or two of smiles, something extra will be done for them that they like)

Eating: Offer what you feel is a healthy meal with a little starch. If child eats starch and walks away, that's fine. No discussion. But when child comes back one hour later hungry, play dumb and serve the leftover food. When not eating well, don't let child snack or have juice in between meals. They need X amount of calories per day no matter where they get it.

Education: If in a special-needs class, try to have some time in a regular class for "normal" role models. Learn to use the computer academically. Work with child fifteen to twenty minutes on computer, then the child can have thirty to forty minutes to do something they enjoy. The computer (and age-appropriate programs) can be a wonderful tool to review developmental steps orderly, logically, but is best if integrated into steps to help a child generalize (whatever is being taught on the computer, etc.), fill in, and understand the gaps they missed.

Speech: Need speech pathologist who can redevelop skills that were missed and who also is familiar with oral apraxia. Think of a stressed/injured brain (like that of a stroke victim) that needs rehabilitation.

Sleep: If child has trouble sleeping or falling asleep, talk to the child and explain that when it is dark outside, they need to stay in bed, let their brain rest. Even if you can't sleep, you need to lie there and rest. If child comes out of his or her room, you then need a control point;, i.e,: lock on the outside of the door, no nightlight, etc. If child will stay in room, then nightlight will be allowed to stay on, etc. Goal is for child to stay in bed and rest (will usually fall asleep) even if they can't sleep.

Siblings: Try to help a brother or sister understand their brother / sister has been ill, and they can become a part of helping them get better. Siblings can be the best therapists.

11

THE FUTURE

W E HAVE WITNESSED THE EVOLUTION OF what is now being recognized and accepted at the National Institutes of Health (NIH), the Centers for Disease Control (CDC), and academic institutions worldwide as a "neuroimmune" epiphenomenon. Studies are now confirming the concept of physiologic immune-mediated diseases underlying an abnormal physiologic state for these patients. This, in turn, creates both physical and neurocognitive deficits and dysfunction, usually of long-term duration. The ongoing failure to "connect the dots," understand the true magnitude of the medical epidemic we are facing, as noted previously, is beyond understanding or comprehension.

I believe that many of the characteristics ascribed to autistic (and "quiet" ADHD) children overlap with the multiple complaints of adults afflicted with components of CFS/CFIDS and adult "ADHD." As previously noted, all of these groups have reports of various immune abnormalities including T cell changes reflected, for example, by increased or decreased CD4/CD8 cells, increased/decreased NK and B cells, and altered viral titers. It is this common denominator of immune alterations that gives hope for potential new therapies in the near future for these children. However, while this hypothesis now has support in the literature, there are many important questions to be answered. How many "autistic" children have evidence of or are linked to an immune-dysfunctional state or a conclusive viral etiology? Can these children be viewed and treated differently than the "classic autistic" child of twenty to thirty years ago? Is their prognosis for recovery significantly better than the "classic autistic" children from the past? It is time to recognize that these children are likely suffering from a medical disease process and need our clinical and research efforts now! Current treatments need to be modified and adjusted to account for this finding. The symptoms of the "quiet" ADD child (who is likely connected to this phenomenon) is not consistent with the past training or processes used to "explain" and address the "hyper" ADD child. It seems likely that the cognitive defects described in adults and children with CFIDS may be thought of as milder, later-onset form of "autism" (really NIDS) as they are similar in symptomatology and possible etiologies. The continued exploration of an immune-dysfunctional epiphenomenon, and the potential etiologies linked to it, is a door we must walk through if we expect to change the future of this generation of children! If a child is born developmentally miswired, "damaged," something happened in utero. But a child cannot learn to speak and use language and then lose these abilities if the cause of their disorder is developmental or structural. Such a child cannot respond to treatment and become a regular child once more, as has been the case in my practice over and over again, if the cause of their disorder is a "fixed" process, congenital or genetic disorder. It has been repeatedly apparent that four-, five-, six-year-old children are starting over where they left off at eighteen months, two years of age. Parents who were told their children would never talk, could never be social, could never have feelings, now have children who are functioning normally or who are still struggling to catch up. In either case these parents can see or are beginning to see a future for their child. We must focus our efforts on saving this generation of children before it is too late. The ramifications are enormous. At the end of a research symposium in October 1997 that brought together top researchers from around the country to discuss Alzheimer's, adult dementias, social brain, and autism/pervasive developmental disorder (PDD), this statement was made: If a child developed normally during the first twelve, fifteen, eighteen months of life, developed any language/words, and then somehow went into this autistic spectrum, it was a 100 percent certainty that the process had to be immune/viral. If a child developed normally the first twelve, fifteen, eighteen months of life and had *no* words, 99 percent it was an immune/viral process, and no one there could rationalize any other possible mechanism. While there is ongoing controversy regarding past brain biopsy findings and their implications, if any, to this generation of children, we do have NeuroSPECT scans, which show reproducible, quantifiable blood flow in the brain. Blood flow corresponds directly to function. When NeuroSPECT scans of children diagnosed as autistic/PDD have been correlated with MRIs and CAT scans, the combination consistently shows no preexisting damage to the brain, but rather points toward an immune mediated shutdown consistent with that found in adults with chronic fatigue syndrome and other adult dementias and with children diagnosed as quiet ADD and mixed ADD. Paralleling this, beginning in the 1980s was the initially slow, now epidemic incidence of disorders in children labeled as autism/PDD and the increase of reports of autoimmune diseases in the animal literature, of altered ecological balance, immune system abnormalities in various species. We either have to assume that this increase of disorders in the human population is mass hysteria, mass psychosis, mass schizophrenia, and/or an impossible epidemic of behavioral developmental disorders in children or we must step back and realize that maybe we have a large number of adults and children suffering from a disease process that is affecting how their brain and nervous system functions, in ways that physicians had never understood (or had the technology to understand). I have family after family within my "new" practice in which there is a mother or father with chronic fatigue syndrome, an older child with ADD/ADHD, and a younger child or two with autism/PDD. As noted, unless we assume this is all random, there is unfortunately a logical connection between the above disorders and their rapid emergence as a crisis. We are looking at what appears, supported by increasing data and reports in the literature, to be autoimmune, neuroimmune disorders or what my associates and I have termed neuro immune dysfunction syndromes or NIDS. If you are an adult with an intelligent, developed brain or an older teenager, when this process attacks, you will likely end up being diagnosed with the illnesses such as chronic fatigue syndrome, adult ADHD, etc. If you are a younger child, five, six, seven, or eight years old when this process is triggered, with some cognitive, social, and language capabilities already developed, you will likely develop what is called quiet ADD or mixed ADD. If you are twelve, fifteen, eighteen months old, however, when this process begins, you will have barely begun to develop cognitive, language, and social skills and you will wind up with what has been called autism/PDD.

The good news is that this concept is supported by commonsense medical logic. The bad news is that we must unify and focus efforts or we will continue to see more adults that are supposed to be paying taxes and earning a living finding themselves on welfare, unable to function, unable to produce. Even graver is that if nothing changes, we are currently raising an entire generation of children to this fate (and worse).

There is *hope*. Research from many prominent institutions supports the idea that the brain is pliable at least into adolescence, and early adulthood, possibly even beyond. It has been my rewarding experience as a pediatrician to see five-year-olds, eight-year-olds, ten-year-olds, and even a twelve-year-old boy who could not talk, begin to use language. Parents, who were told their child would never be independent, never able to earn a living, and who one day might have to be placed in an institution, have seen their children become top of their class academically. I have children within the practice scoring in the 97th, even the 99th percentile on California and Illinois state testing.

We must bring together physicians and pediatric subspecialists, speech pathologists, educational specialists, and "rehab" specialists. While many present "experts" may be "out of work," there is an immediate need to mobilize and train many experts who know how to help redevelop and redesign programs to mazimize the potential of each of these children. We must make this happen while moving rapidly to improve brain and body functioning for these children, medically, logically, safely.

The potential multiple triggers for this illness we call NIDS will need many, many years of ongoing research to learn how multiple factors including stress, viral infection, or environmental contaminants may play a role. The key is to focus treatment efforts, rapidly, effectively—*now*—to keep from losing an entire generation of children while the ultimate "answers" are still being investigated. We can use technology to accurately define "subgroups" of these children and adults. Discussion appearing recently in the pediatric literature that up to 25 percent of neurotypical, "healthy" children have some type of chronic disorder, characterized by allergies, migraines, asthma, and diabetes should be one of those earth-shattering calls to action by our pediatric societies and those involved in many areas with helping parents and their children. Where would we be today if most of us grew up in a society saying 25 percent of "normal" children already had long-term chronic illness. The negative implication socially and medically should be staggering. This should mobilize an immediate call for answers, not just reexploration of theories that have never fully explained or accounted for this now staggering number of children and adolescents.

Confirming the general ideas linked above, another article that should have increased overall focus and concern was a publication in *Pediatrics* in October 2008,[1] confirming a significant increase of allergic and immune abnormalities in children with complex medical problems. Not psychiatric, not developmental, immune. The report confirmed along with altered immune markers and reactions to cow's milk and other antigens, these patients often had various gastroesophageal disorders, failure to thrive, sleep disturbances, and recurrent otitis media. The author reported on "a higher than expected prevalence of allergic and immune abnormalities in children with complex medical problems."

Perhaps this should lead to an increased urgency to review and look at concepts in this book, open the doors to addressing new ways to perhaps dramatically improve a child's condition of life, even if the "NIDS" component is not the whole answer or reason for the disorder, it is a potentially treatable aspect today.

The ideas presented in this book of what should be done in therapy to help a child become healthier, redevelop their abilities, and function is based on this being an illness. It remains unfortunate that the vast majority of the medical and therapeutic world—physicians, therapists, educators—are led to believe, somehow, in a "mysterious" manner, these children are born damaged, somehow miswired, somehow something has gone wrong "developmentally."

There is *no* objective evidence supporting a diagnosis of "autism," most ideas of "ADHD," and yet we just assume things are this way. In reality, all objective evidence supports the information being presented in this book, the idea that there is some type of a "complex neuroimmune, complex viral" disease process occurring.

Therapies have been aimed at trying to help, while focusing mostly on behaviors, control, and all too often "training" a presumably "autistic" child. Automatically, with the recognition of the fact these children are ill, this is not the fastest growing developmental disorder ever, then therapeutically you cannot treat them different, do things to them that you would not do to support or help any other potentially "neurotypically" normal child. The academic world, instead of looking at application of antipsychotics or anticonvulsants, will have to focus on therapies against the disease process itself, other therapies to help these children cognitively. "Alternative medicine" will either have to validate its true safety, efficacy, or it will not be allowed to be done. Many therapists practicing alternative medicine are more than aware of what this would mean. This discussion has tremendous implications for debates about therapy. As much as I may not like it, one can argue if one thinks a child is miswired, brain damaged, then some type of "dog training" is better than nothing at all. If one understands these are not previously damaged children, certainly as soon as you begin to get that glimmer of a brighter brain, one must think of appropriate techniques to rehabilitate that child. As a physician, as a scientist, you debate what comes first, the chicken or the egg? The immune system or virus? It appears over many decades now that immune system dysfunction is going to be the key, and is likely the first area of dysfunction, with viruses secondary, acting opportunistically. It is safe to say that 100 percent of these patients have "neuroimmune dysfunction." Many more seem to have viral issues now than in the early years of looking at this phenomenon. While this physician's opinion is that the viruses remain secondary, not the primary reason for this; that statement must be open to new research, the potential discovery of some unknown pathogen, some unknown virus underneath all this. As I was taught in high school, college, and then medical school, we live in a sea of viruses; we are surrounded by viruses with which we have learned how to coexist in an equilibrium; but when we become ill, when our immune systems are not there to protect us fully, these viruses can become significant pathogens. Note: This concept is perhaps best illustrated by the original sci-fi classic *War of the Worlds*. In the book, in the terrifying radio broadcast of 1939, what stopped the Martian invaders? The common cold virus. With no build in immunity, the lesson was, even the common cold could kill you. A true statement! Almost like the Martians, are our children being undone and our society eventually toppled by in this case a combination of microorganisms, and our now stressed, dysfunctional immune systems? Under the frequent misdirection of psychiatry, our sophistication but complete lack of recognition of the real problem is leaving us all open, our children most vulnerable, to this debilitating, potentially life-threatening process. We are not controlling a potential attack of pathogens we lived with for thousands of years, and by mistake our own immune systems think "we're a foreign organism—a Martian." I believe that if we focus on the right things, we have the resources and the ability to fight back and win this battle. Before it's too late, please join in.

In Summary

With the bleak prospects for a child diagnosed with autism perpetuated by academics and alternative medicine, one cannot blame a parent for being encouraged by any glimmer of hope. Many of the remedies are likely to cause harm over time, and perhaps that is why so few children maintain what is at times considered good progress to begin with. In terms of "autism" expectations are kept low; in terms of the reality of an "illness" parents should have a right to have high expectations. No longer could "academics" or "alternative" medicine prescribe pharmaceutical agents or supplements, or recommend procedures that will likely cause long-term harm to a potentially normal child or child's brain.

All of the connections and family relationships do not make sense in any simple terms of genetics or developmental, but rather, only in the context of a slowly expanding, medical epidemic. This epidemic is acting in an insidious manner, unlike what most epidemiologists or medical professionals are taught to think about when it comes to infectious disease, much less any remote idea of an "immune related" epidemic.

These children present with a *symptomatology* consisting primarily of severe speech and language development (left temporal lobe) and severe social difficulties (right temporal lobe), often some fine, not usually gross, motor difficulties (cerebellar involvement), and various learning difficulties and attention deficit dysfunctions consistent with involvement of frontal and temporal lobes, and sometimes its links to areas of parietal-occipital dysfunction.

They may also have many symptoms consistent with OCD and ADHD characteristics, associated with these areas of dysfunction.

As noted, in adolescents and adults, this dysfunction may manifest itself as CFIDS (chronic fatigue immune dysfunction syndrome), ADHD "variants," and various other atypical autoimmune disorders associated with neuroimmune dysfunction. In older children, it is seen as variants of ADD (attention deficit disorder)/ADHD. And in younger children/ infants, it appears as autism/ autistic syndrome/PDD. If we continue to ignore the now-obvious connection and the bigger picture, what will happen to our society, economic, and social system ultimately around the world (already in a state of stress, needless to say). When at least 25 percent of neurotypical children have chronic illnesses (including diabetes, obesity, allergies, migraines, asthma)—what is going to happen as these children grow up? I have never been exposed to any teaching in college or medical school that says our society, or any society, can handle that many citizens with chronic illness/disease. I cannot conceive of going into pediatric training and being told that 25 percent of my patients were going to be chronically ill (and that I couldn't change that!).

Since the "system" has not woken up (or is waking up as slowly as it can), the issue facing many readers of this book, all parents out there, is what can be done now, what can be done to change the future for their child maybe tomorrow, not in another decade or longer. Parents must come together as they have not done before.

It has become obvious that over the years, many errors, misdirections in research have occurred, but looking back, the mistakes have occurred in spite of good intentions by contributors and parents. We all grew up, and I was trained with a strong belief in our "ivory towers." As echoed in the Hollywood community, in theory this was the era in which "there was no disease we couldn't solve with enough funding." It is obvious to me and to many frantic parents by now that our "ivory towers," the main medical focus led by psychiatrists (as noted, these disorders as defined decades ago were not considered to have primary medical issues/problems), and all the money to date, have not remotely helped solve the real crisis, a true medical crisis facing these children and adults. The situation is so bad, so controlled, that I have been told multiple times that in major institutions, if you want to study developmental or genetics, you will likely be funded (look at all the money raised, and added to this system by congress and private support groups), but if you want to study immune or viral, not only should you not expect funding, but you may be reprimanded (bad judgment if not a very high up researcher) or even let go. Somehow, that does not resemble the medical or academic world I was exposed to or have believed in.

A second major point of misdirections and lack of focus for parents is living in a world where the Internet is fact. While misstatements, misinterpretations, and outright lies apply to all fields and all areas of information discussed on the Internet, this has had a particulary devastating affect within the field of medicine, where parents want to believe what they read (but while how to dissect, understand a medical article is part of Medical School 101—it is not part of basic training for parents or patients.)

In the past (i.e., polio, measles, or other serious childhood illness), when multiple children were being hit by an illness, when parents were living under constant threat of a serious illness affecting their children, they became a part of the solution by demanding mobilization of the medical and pharmaceutical world to help their children fight these terrifying epidemics. Today, parents frustrated about a lack of scientific evidence, tests, and research, and who are desperate to help their children, are embracing "alternative" medicine which offers glimpses of improvement (based on multiple anecdotal, completely noncontrolled reports on the Internet). The "alternative" medicine system has been so vocal, but often so misdirected, that their ongoing distribution of proposed mechanisms and ideas (some possible, most *not*), have only helped misdirect a system already starting from a confused, dysfunctional place. As a pediatrician trained to review data and controlled studies, I have yet to see a controlled trial of any kind validating what is being proposed by most alternative medicine physicians (beyond parent or internet support), and worse, after fifteen-plus years— where are the long-term success stories from these other ideas or protocols? This author continues to remain skeptical of any therapy or claims that do not *begin* with clinical and physiologic logic, real potential efficacy or safety based on the real pathophysiology of these disorders.

With the obvious neuroimmune linkages to Alzheimer's, Parkinson's, and schizophrenia (and likely many other adult and child dementias), how can we continue to ignore a major pathway that could help so many patients? By studying each of these areas as their own problem, we are opening missing a major direction that not only will likely unify a large group of these patients, especially those that are called "atypical," but also could lead rapidly to new approaches of therapy, likely far more successful than what's been done for decades, for many suffering today. We have evolved to a system that is so specialized, so focused on minutia, that we have lost sight of the bigger picture, the potential bigger connection. Research goes on in the United States, Europe continuing to focus on variations of rheumatoid diseases, variations of autism and autism spectrum, variations of ADHD, and other learning disorders, variants of lupus, Alzheimer's, MS, and other related autoimmune disorders, the list goes on and on.

What if there are so many variants of each of these disorders because many of the variants and classic presentations are really part of a bigger picture, a bigger disease pathway of "complex neuroimmune, complex viral diseases."

As illustrated by the slow progress for so many of these chronic disorders, if we wait till we understand every fine detail of each dysfunction, if we wait for the "holy grail" (the ability to engineer enough genes that we might alter or change some of these disorders), we are going to continue to fail these patients and their families. The current rates of illness (1:110 children with autism, 1:10 children with ADHD) could conceivably put such strain on government systems and our healthy population as to cause a collapse of society (leaving behind many wealthy researchers, institutes, alternative medicine clinics, and therapists).

This line of thought (acting on what we know and embracing proactive solutions) applies to all diseases including cancers. How long can we study variants of cancers, subcauses, genetics, variations of attempts at therapy to either "cut it out" or destroy the cancer (without destroying the host—the patient)—without addressing the contributions of stress on the body's immune system? By recognizing the negative effects of a stressed immune system, the effects of the environment, and multiple other factors we're exposed to, the common denominator, recognized and discussed at an NIH-sponsored meeting in 1992, is that when our immune systems are stressed, when what are called our NK (Natural Killer) cells are low, we are all prone to chronic viral activations, the risk of cancers, etc. Our bodies naturally produce dysfunctional, cancerous cells quite often, but thankfully most of us stay healthy. Our immune systems were designed to protect us. While many researchers are pursuing ideas of how to use our immune system to try to fight a cancer, maybe it's time to focus on prevention, avoiding that cancer in the first place.

We live in a unique environment. We live our lives on earth and are protected by the ozone layer above us. If the ozone layer becomes damaged, as it has been in the last twenty–thirty years because of man-made stressors and compounds, science says we become bombarded by dangerous UV rays that can damage our bodies. Our brain's immune systems are now under attack in a similar way. Whether it's environmental stressors, a genetically predisposed susceptibility, viruses in hiding, or a combination of these factors—the brains of our children are not healthy. The damage can take years to become evident. It is evident now. And it's the responsibility of the medical community to take action.

For additonal information please visit www.neuroimmunedr.com and www.NIDS.net.

APPENDIX A

○ ○ ○ ◎ ◎ ○ ○ ○

A CASE STUDY

W HEN JENNY FIRST CAME TO ME, and this is typical of about half a
dozen children in the practice, she didn't have any other markers
I was looking at as showing that her immune system was activated, some
of the things I would look for normally as a virus. But she had one very
important one. Her ANA was 1:640 before I even met her. Somehow this
was tested, and nobody did a thing.

By the time I graduated from UCLA, I'd learned that "autoimmune
disorders" were things that happened commonly in adults. These were the
early days of collagen vascular disease, rheumatoid diseases, and lupus.
The characteristic was that these patients did not often have a physical
diagnosis—they didn't have a set disease. However, medicine said this was
abnormal to have an elevated ANA, and these adults were treated as having
a disorder—a disease. Why we can't give the children the same benefit of
the doubt is beyond me.

Jenny's parents were told she was autistic, so what about her ANA?
When I met her, we repeated her value and her ANA was still elevated,
but the rest of her blood work was not particularly exciting. As I do with
most children, I took her off milk, dairy, chocolate, and whole wheat. Her
parents will acknowledge that if she cheats and has a pizza or dairy product,
her behavior becomes off the wall.

I started her on an antifungal, Nizoral. The parents already had her
on low-dose supplements of N-dimethylglycine (DMG), a food substance
found in the cells of the body.

She began to talk a little more. Within a short time I put her on a
selective serotonin reuptake inhibitor (SSRI), which is a compound
typically used as an antidepressant. She began to pick up on her speech
and was interacting better.

As we went along, we introduced another antifungal. She began to lose some of her "autistic" behaviors. We changed her SSRI to Prozac and repeated a little bit of her blood work. Her ANA, at least as a marker, was coming down. She was still showing signs of allergy with her high eosinophils, but the parents felt this child was improving daily.

By August (a month later), her auditory processing was up; her social skills were up. She was not sick anymore. The parents were obviously very happy. In December, their statement to me was that she was doing excellent. She was on amphotericin and Prozac. In her case, she did well with a little bit of echinacea. She still had behavioral issues.

I want to stress this point because this is something that has really become apparent over the years. Many parents would have been thrilled to have this child functioning at the level she was, but what I'm really looking for now is that cognitive functioning. She was having behavioral issues at home and school because she had never grown through the normal social stages.

It became obvious to the parents and teachers that what they were looking at were behavioral situations. But this child, cognitively, was doing extremely well. Jenny even toilet trained.

Why should she suddenly be able to toilet train after years of being unable? I've always been taught as a pediatrician that you don't rush your child on toilet training. When they are ready, they will learn. This same thing is happening with these children as their brain turns back on, starts moving from that fifteen- to eighteen-month-old to two-year-old to two-and-a-half-year-old level, at some point the child toilet trains like any other child.

We bounced her around a little bit on the antifungals with the idea that the amphotericin was probably not holding her. In 1997, again, she kept doing better day by day. She reached a point where she was doing very well by many, many criteria. But it takes years for the brain to evolve. It can't jump from birth to five or birth to ten. These children have to pick up and learn.

By the following June the parents state she is acting more and more "normal." We added an antiviral not because she gave me any viral titers, but because by then it had become apparent that many of these children seem to be fighting a background herpes or retrovirus-type process.

Whether it's because their immune systems are stressed, weakened a little bit, and they are more susceptible to these viruses lasting longer, it is not clear. Within five days, the parents saw a significant improvement; motor skills improved, she became more social, and she made a complaint to her teacher that she could not think at times because her brain hurt.

As she progressed the headaches went away. She seemed to go through cycles of growth like any other child—things will be going well, and they'll seem to plateau, or have a rough drop and then move forward.

By the end of the year she was starting to wake up rested. Whether children are getting enough sleep is a very big factor when I determine whether to treat a child with attention deficit disorder, chronic fatigue syndrome, or autism/PDD. I learned in the late 1980s studying chronic fatigue syndrome at the University of California, Irvine, that when your brain was affected with these illnesses, you did not go into a normal sleep cycle. Researchers documented that these adults with an unknown (at that time) presumably psychiatric disorder were going into a stage where they did not enter normal stage 4 REM sleep cycles. You could sleep eight hours, ten hours, twelve hours and still wake up tired. The end goal is for the patient to wake up feeling rested.

By then, Jenny was going to be in a school play (which she did very well in, by the way). I have many reports from parents in my practice who report that after months of treatments their child took part in their first baseball game or performed in their first school play. That's not something you're told to expect out of your children—but it's possible. As we progressed, we switched her medication to Zoloft. Even though this child had been doing very, very well, the parents came in and said she was doing even bettert.

Let's go back to her diagnosis of autism. This was how she was labeled. I will guarantee you that she does not meet any of those criteria at this point.

Case Study for "H.C.": DOB 5/93

- Large head—could not get down birth canal
- Jaundice
- Limited success with breast feeding—then formula

- Enjoyed interacting with mom and dad
- Some words at 9 months
- At about 1 yr.—whole milk
- Realized not developing language as she should
- Sometimes refuses to cooperate
- National Naval Medical Center—possible "storage problem" in head—decision—nothing abnormal
- Didn't potty train
- Lab: Jenny
- 11/98 ANA—Neg
- HHV6 IGG <20
- CD4 1180
- CD8 502
- NK Cells 8 percent
- *Interferon alpha:* 439
- Gliadin—Neg.
- Folate 11.7
- Vit. B12—911.4
- 3/00 ferritin—43
- 3/01 HHV6 IGG 1:80
- CD4 1144
- CD8 506
- NK Cells 5.0 percent
- 5/01 interferon alpha <5
- ASO—695

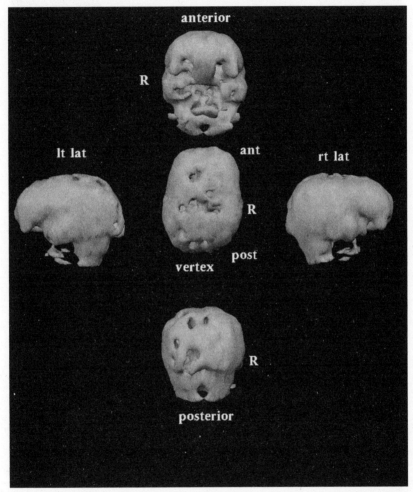

Initial 3-D NeuroSPECT imaging on patient "H.C." "Holes" are multiple areas of decreased perfusion and decreased function in the brain. This brain scan graphically illustrates the difficulty of normal brain function when "holes" are present.

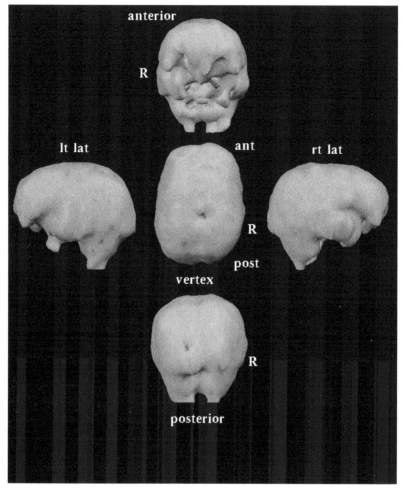

NeuroSPECT scan 2.5 years later, after treatment with The Goldberg Approach (see chapter 7). While brain function is not normal, it is significantly improved.

Conclusion: this disorder and its complications can be changed.

APPENDIX B

○ ○ ◎ ◉ ◎ ○ ○

PARENT STORIES

"Ryan"

As parents we belong to a very unique group, the A-club, where only the chosen, crazy, and determined can survive the autism diagnosis. None of us ever wanted to join the autism club, or ever asked to become members. But, because of our kids we were all forced to be in it together. Only another parent understands what it is like to live with this diagnosis day in and day out. The isolation and loneliness this diagnosis brings can be overwhelming. The hardest part is to continue to get up every day and not give up on our kids. What if everything we read or were told about autism is not necessarily true? What if what we are talking about is not a debilitating psychiatric disorder without any hope for recovery? What if it is a medical condition caused in most part by an immune system that is not working properly? What if autism is treatable? My kid recovered and was kicked out of the A-club because of the medical treatment he received from Dr. Goldberg, a doctor who was ahead of his time. I want all your kids to be kicked out too.

Ryan was diagnosed when he was four by the leading authority on autism in the Twin Cities. She told us my son would never be okay and would probably end up in a group home or institution. When my son entered kindergarten at almost six years old, he was in the 3rd percentile for speech. By that time Dr. Goldberg had been treating Ryan medically for about a year. Ryan had a full-time aide in his classroom to help him in school. By the third grade, my son tested in the 85th percentile for speech, and by fifth grade Ryan no longer received any services or assistance at school.

As a result of the medical treatment from Dr. Goldberg, the only institution Ryan is in today is the university he currently attends on a merit-based academic scholarship. Ryan does all the things the doctors told me he would never do.

He studies mechanical engineering and is number two in his class. He joined the Sigma Chi fraternity and is president of the Jewish Student Association. Ryan drives, has a ton of friends, and even has a girlfriend. (Who would have seen that one coming?) But more important, Ryan is happy. If anyone would have told me this was possible when he was little, I never would have believed them. Unbelievable as it seems, this is the same child who wanted to spend his days plugging a portable radio into every outlet in the house over and over again. Ryan is an example of what is possible for children with autism when they receive proper medical and behavioral interventions. They can grow up to lead productive and happy lives.

Ryan's long road to recovery was the hardest thing I have ever lived through. I remember questioning if my family's sacrifices and efforts were accomplishing anything. I wasn't sure if I had the strength to be more stubborn than my son. There were mornings I didn't want to get out of bed just to face another day filled with autism. The worst times were when I didn't have a direction or a plan. I was just hanging on by my fingernails. But, at the end of the day, I was faced with a choice: let Ryan drift off forever into his own world, or drag him kicking and screaming into ours.

After Dr. Goldberg addressed Ryan's medical problems, it took years to correct Ryan's deficits in speech and social skills. Behavioral and educational interventions were needed to help him catch up. Everything he missed while he was autistic had to be taught. The weird behaviors and habits he developed to cope had to be eliminated. It was almost like bringing back a stroke victim.

Those of us who have lived with an autistic child understand the daily struggles associated with our out-of-control kids. We know how putting on a pair of shoes can cause a major confrontation or getting a child into the car can be more than exhausting. The enormous cost associated with the medical, behavioral, and educational treatments for autism is just another obstacle we must overcome.

The kind of medical intervention that Dr. Goldberg provides needs to become common knowledge and what every doctor can do for children with autism. When that happens, we will learn just how "possible" recovery can be for these seemingly "impossible" children. We must not give up on our children no matter how difficult the road becomes or how hard our children try to make us give up. We have work to do to make the world and the medical communities understand that what our children are facing is not a psychiatric disorder but rather a treatable medical immune problem. My hope is that what happened for Ryan becomes the norm rather than the exception. Something must be done, because there are kids *not* getting better every day.

"Michael"

Michael was always a very sweet and handsome little boy. He always smiled and really had very few wants. He loved watching videos and was very content to play with the things he loved. He didn't really have much language, but since he was the third child and a boy, we figured he was on his own time line. As he started to get older, around two years of age, he still wasn't responding to his name, and he was just muttering some "ma ma, da da" syllables. At his first and second birthdays, he didn't respond when asked to come and sing "Happy Birthday." He was also preoccupied with lining up train tracks and staring at the wheels of his little school bus and car figures. We would call out his name and got no response. I would ask who wanted to go for ice cream, and my girls would be screaming with excitement, and Michael just looked at me cluelessly as if he were a child that was just brought over from Russia. Soon it became apparent that there was something *very* wrong! My friends thought he might be deaf, but I wasn't really sure what was going on. I knew he heard me, since I sang to him all the time and he gave me the sweetest smiles a mom could ever ask for. He only responded to me and barely knew his grandparents and other family members and friends that loved him and wanted so much to be a part of this beautiful boy's life.

So, time to take him to the neurologist in N.Y.C. I think this was the worst day of my life! I was told that Michael had PDD and that this was something that would be extremely difficult to deal with. I was told to start speech therapy immediately and to do my best. The scary thing is that I didn't even know what this PDD was. All I knew was Dustin Hoffman in *Rain Man.* I was quite unfamiliar with the word "autism," and I really didn't know how I was going to be able to deal with this. Michael was two and three months at the time. Well, after I almost had a nervous breakdown my incredible husband told me it was time to stop feeling sorry for myself and time to take care of myself, my three kids, and our family. I seriously jumped into action and started speech therapy and early intervention and worked like a dog to try and keep Michael engaged and to teach him how to become a person. Michael made some nice improvements from the time of diagnosis to the age of 4½ but not enough for me. He was still only using three–four word sentences, and he was still very much involved in his own world unless I pulled him out. We also used ABA as well as speech therapy, and I had him involved in a mainstream nursery school as well. But again, Michael wasn't making the gains that I knew he could, so it was time for a change!

I got Dr. Goldberg's name from a teacher who spoke very highly of him and told me that when I was ready for drastic changes in Michael's life, it was the time for Dr. G. She told me he would need major blood work and would have to go on a special diet and begin taking medicine on a daily basis. Truthfully, I was so scared but I was *desperate*! I needed Michael to get better, and I just knew he was too young to just be given up on. Thus began our journey with Dr. Goldberg. Michael began with Dr. Goldberg at the age of five, and he is now seventeen. It's so interesting how things start becoming so obvious when looking back. The first thing I realized is that Michael only ate and craved dairy before Dr. G. He would eat three or four yogurts at a time, and it seemed that with each yogurt he became more like a "drunken bum." All these foods put Michael into a bigger fog than he started in and it is amazing to me how I didn't realize this until years after seeing how different Michael became after being taken off. I know this to be true since Michael was caught a few times eating yogurt and you could tell almost immediately that something was consumed that shouldn't have been. This really was incredible. Who would ever have thought that dairy could be such a bad thing for a young child? Well, I learned *a lot* from Dr. Goldberg, and I changed everything in Michael's life. No more dairy and foods that were not considered "safe" for Michael, no more allowing Michael to be anything but his best, no more letting people think Michael was "disabled" but teaching them that Michael had a serious illness, and we were working really hard to help him to recover. Everyone in my family along with my closest friends jumped on board to help me with anything I asked them to do. I just did what Dr. G. told me to do and lived through the ups and downs of trying to move Michael forward. The early years were not easy, and there were a lot of tears but there was a lot of joy too! Dr. G. told me I needed to be patient, work hard, and look at Michael's condition as a medical illness and together we would find a way to help Michael get healthy. Well, Michael worked very hard as did we all, and little by little he started making nice improvements—slowly but surely! He started talking better, began trying new foods, and joined our world at times. Each day was a challenge, but we went from so many days of sadness and frustration to small incremental steps of happiness. Sometimes Michael took three steps back, but then he leaped four steps forward. I really began understanding the importance of keeping to the diet and taking the medicine as directed. I really witnessed what happened if Michael cheated on the diet or I forgot to give him his meds. What a powerful pull these two combinations had on Michael's body and brain. WE were also doing intensive therapy and really teaching Michael the rules of life, whether he wanted to learn them or not. Dr. Goldberg was a wonderful, caring doctor and friend throughout this process, and I am extremely thankful that he came into Michael's life (as well as mine!). Michael also had two brain spec scans at the request of Dr. Goldberg so he could really see what was going on in Michael's brain and figure out what medical changes might be necessary to help Michael move forward. All I can say is that I feel that Michael would not be where he is had he not been a patient of Dr. Goldberg's. Michael has made such incredible strides over the years. He went from being a nonverbal child, living in his own world with no clue about anything in life, to a young man who is so capable of so many things. Michael is still a sweet and caring young man who is an active part of our world. Dr. Goldberg gave me hope at a time where top neurologists at Columbia Presbyterian in N.Y. were telling me to do my best but the prognosis wasn't great. The day I met Dr. Goldberg was the last day I *ever* contacted a neurologist again! Michael is now a handsome, sweet young man who has an opinion; who gets to school on his own; navigates through his classes; enjoys being with friends; loves tennis, biking, and basketball; and adores his family. He is loved by all, and he just has a passion for life. He is such a gift, and I find it so incredibly scary to think that there are so many other kids out there with potential who weren't lucky enough to have a doctor like Dr. Goldberg who believes that what has been commonly diagnosed as autism today is a medical condition that can be changed. I love this child and I get goose bumps on a daily basis thinking about all the things Michael has been able to overcome as he has gotten healthier. When I get upset with Michael for something and he says he's sorry, I ask him why he thinks I am upset, and he always says, "I know, Mom, 'cause you want me to be the best kid I can be. I know what I have to do and I will try harder tomorrow." Then a big kiss and we are on to the next topic. I will *never* take talking for granted as long as I live. What a gift. I thank Dr. Goldberg for making Michael's body and brain function better so he can enjoy all the things life has to offer. Looking forward to the next few years! Can't wait to see all the wonderful things still ahead of Michael.

"Eric"

Eric was adopted at birth. He was a wonderful baby who developed normally and had great language up until nineteen months old. By his second birthday, he wasn't responding to his name or using more than one word. He also went from being incredibly happy to distracted and difficult to manage. While my pediatrician assured me that boys develop slower, I knew something was wrong.

The initial diagnosis of the "A" word came from a neurologist at the University of Wisconsin–Madison. We disagreed with him and continued our search for information. We visited numerous other medical centers, and a potential death sentence came from Kennedy Krieger at Johns Hopkins in November of 1999. After two days of testing and thousands of dollars, they told us Eric was severely mentally retarded with *no* capacity to learn. Part of their recommendation was for us to start searching for group homes. While we were shocked at this diagnosis, we didn't accept it. We had seen Eric in action, a problem solver, bright and inquisitive. Instead we continued to seek out other medical advice and opportunities. We were introduced to a DAN doctor who suggested supplements and Kirkman Labs powder since Eric's immune system was compromised and this protocol would help. Eric went crazy—impossible to reason with, compulsive, erratic. So to work through this until his immune system "evened out," this DAN doctor prescribed increasing doses of Neurontin and starting chelation. Our life was insane. Eric never slept and was a constant aggressive mess. We knew his brain was being fried and this clearly wasn't the right path. We were done with the DAN doctor since sessions of chelation was out of the question for us. While we continued with school, speech and language therapy, and OT, we weren't making a lot of progress. Then, in the summer of 2002, we received a call from a friend who lives in Los Angeles. She had seen an article about Dr. G. in the *Los Angeles Times*. Although the journey since meeting Dr. G. in January 2003 has been long, Eric is doing amazingly well. His initial NeuroSPECT showed excess blood flow to the front temporal lobes and many hot spots. His follow-up spec three years later showed a much healthier brain! Years later, he has great language, is in a public high school walking the halls and functioning well. He is calm and focused with the help of tutors and hours of educational interventions. While our journey is far from over, Eric would never have a chance at a life without Dr. G. and his medical interventions.

"Joshua"

Joshua was born April 5, 1996. This was the most wonderful day of our lives. My husband and I had been married for ten years, and we were so ready for the challenges of parenthood. I had the most perfect pregnancy and was healthy the entire time. When Joshua was born, he was the most beautiful baby. My friends were so jealous because they would say he was the perfect baby. He didn't fuss much and was so happy. When Joshua was one year old, I started a business out of my home so I could be with him. We hired a part-time nanny who spoke some English and Spanish. By Joshua's eighteen-month wellness checkup, I remember the doctor was impressed with his speech. He had hit every milestone up to that point. I only remember Joshua getting sick one time as an infant. He had a high fever, and he was taking amoxicillin. I was out of town when my husband called and said Joshua had developed a rash over his torso. We came to believe that he was allergic to the medicine. We later discovered that he was not allergic to penicillin but possibly had contracted the roseola virus. This would later play a part in what I believe helped develop his condition.

By two years old I noticed Joshua was no longer using the many words he had before. I took him to the pediatrician and they told me not to worry and he was probably processing two languages because the nanny spoke Spanish. By two and a half years old my next-door neighbor, who is a third grade teacher, suggested I take Joshua to be tested with the school district at age three and perhaps I could get some free speech services. I took her suggestion, and the school district psychologist reviewed Joshua over several days. At the end of their evaluation, the two women handed me and my husband a six-page report. I remember reading the report, and my head started spinning. I felt like I was going to pass out. I remember the ladies using the autism word and saying how "some" children can lead full lives and maybe get simple jobs when they are adults. They did remind me that many of these children will most likely need to be cared for the rest of their lives. I felt physically sick, and my whole world and dreams came crashing down. They gave us the standard package with services that were available and funding from RCOC. Because we had waited until Joshua was three years old, we didn't qualify for much and were at the school district's mercy.

When we got home, I remember my husband wasting no time. He started talking to other parents. This ended out being the best thing ever. I find that those who lived through this sort of thing are so full of helpful knowledge about the schools. Back in 1996 this "autism" thing was such a mystery, and though the numbers were beginning to soar (one in five hundred), they were nothing like they are now. Back then you never heard of the "A" word. One parent we spoke to became at the time our guardian angel. She recommended that we not put Joshua in the school district program but develop our own in-home program. She gave us contacts with great therapists and wonderful resources. That woman, Marta, will never fully know the impact she had on our lives. Once the fog cleared up in our brains, we became research junkies. At the time the only hope we saw was in ABA training. Dr. Ivan Lovass from UCLA developed a program that he claimed "cured" this affliction. The key to this treatment was early intervention. We scrambled to try to get Joshua set up with this type of training and found many roadblocks. We faced agencies saying there were up to two-year waiting list. With CARD organization, we were 103 on their list. Out of complete desperation, my husband, Gary, faxed a letter to Dr. Lovass. We found out he was still alive and was running Lovass Institute For Early Intervention (LIFE). Our plea was desperate, and we begged them to consider taking Joshua. Our first miracle came on a Tuesday when a man named Mario contacted us and said that they had availability for an Orange County family. We went to work gathering our head therapist and hiring college students who would be willing to learn this technique. In the next two years, Joshua soared through the program. Within two weeks into the program he was starting to talk again. His progress was so unbelievable, and he seemed to master programs in record time. This treatment was extremely expensive, and my husband and I worked full-time to pay for what I call Joshua's "Harvard" education. These two years were so hard on us financially and even harder on my marriage. It seemed the strain and total focus of our lives were so completely wrapped up in Joshua that my husband and I found ourselves strangers after fourteen years of marriage. I filed for divorce, but God had different plans.

My real miracle: "You don't know God is all you need until God is all you have." That is the place our family found ourselves. Unable on our own to bridge the divide of pain that separated my husband and me, we sought out Christian counseling. God did quick work and my husband and I reconciled. In that process is when we really sought God's direction with our son. We noticed that Joshua had plateaued in the program, and we didn't know how much further we could go with the LIFE program. He was of kindergarten age, and we choose to delay Joshua's enrollment for a year. We were receiving some partial funding for our in-home program, and we felt blessed for that aid. In the meantime in that summer on 2001, I had another child. I was so convinced that God was going to bring a girl in our life. I had been praying for a sister for Joshua so she can take care of him someday and I wouldn't ever have to worry about his future. The odds of having another autistic child with a girl was so much less then with a boy that I was convinced that God would not put me through that again. Well God only gives you what you can handle, and I was having another boy! When I found out, I was devastated. Suddenly the reality that we might have to go through this again was more than I could bear. Although Joshua was doing great and was having many successes, the diagnosis is so all consuming and I realized how tired I was. For two weeks I felt a heavy fear regarding this new baby coming into our life. And one morning I remember a thought coming into my mind. "Do you want to live in fear or faith?" When you live in fear you are allowing the joy of your life to be stolen from you. I remember at that moment that I was going to live by faith. We had a healthy baby Noah on August 5, 2001. At this time I started getting more insight on Joshua. He didn't seem like a typical autistic boy. There was something more. I starting praying, "What else is it, God? What else should we do for Joshua?"

That night the woman who I said was our guardian angel called me. I had not talked to her for two years and she called because she heard about Joshua's great success. She wanted me to talk to a mother about starting an in-home program. Then in almost an afterthought, she mentioned I should call this lady because her son was "healed." I was shocked and got the phone number. I did not know at the time that call would change our lives forever! This lady told me to *stop* what I was doing and go see Dr. Goldberg. I had heard of Dr. Goldberg and didn't know what to expect. She was so insistent, and when we were on the phone her son came on the line asking about a Hot Wheels car he was looking for. I asked if that was her son and she said yes. He sounded so natural, so normal, so alive. I wanted that for my son and I made the appointment. When we got to the doctors, Dr. Goldberg made so much sense, and we did all the blood work needed. When we got the results, Joshua's blood work was very clear. He had the second highest HHV6 (human herpes virus six) count that the doctor had seen. On future research, I believe the virus grew in Joshua from that roseola virus when he was younger. I later found out he was *not* allergic to penicillin. The HHV6 is found in roseola, and it definitely was a contributing factor. When I asked the doctor what he thought Joshua had, he described it as NIDS (neuroimmune dysfunction syndrome). He said it was like a type of "brain virus." The virus hides in the brain and masquerades itself like various afflictions (autism, ADD/ADHD, and chronic fatigue syndrome). We put Joshua on the NIDS protocol, and within sixty days he was unrecognizable. The progress was so amazing that I went back to the school district and insisted that we put Joshua in kindergarten! We believe in the treatment so much we gave back the district $27,000 they approved to help with our home program! They were so shocked by his progress, and I explained to them our findings. Because the district had no time to find an aide for Joshua in the class, they agreed to hire Joshua's two head therapists. From that moment on, Joshua has thrived. He has never set foot in a special-needs class and has had only minimal shadowing and aides in his classes. The IEPs that started out as a battlefield became a venue to discuss Joshua's great progress. My IEPs ended up being praise reports more than anything else! Joshua continued to be one of the brightest students in every class he has ever been in. During the elementary years we focused on social skills and containing emotions. Each year we saw more and more victory in his life. In fifth grade, Joshua really came into his own. He got the lead in the school play, and it skyrocketed his confidence and popularity. He was a straight A student, and the teachers really enjoy his positive attitude.

In sixth grade we were pretty apprehensive about putting him in our public school. It is really large. We completely went without any aide or shadow and cut the umbilical cord. This was a risky move because once you discontinue services, you can't get them back. We had faith in Joshua. Now, Joshua is graduating from the eighth grade in a few weeks, and we could not be prouder of him. He still struggles to keep his allergies in check and with his HHV6 numbers, but with each passing day Joshua is getting healthier. In the three years of junior high he has surpassed everyone's expectations with amazing grades (102 As and 4 Bs). Joshua has developed amazing guitar-playing skills and written and has recorded his first album, *Autosanity*. He will be attending Tesoro High School and has many exciting challenges ahead. His goals are to attend MIT and become an engineer so he can design roller coasters. I believe my son has a bright and successful future and I know that his treatment with Dr. Goldberg has saved his life. Not from death, but from a handicapped life, a debilitating life. He is only fourteen years old!

"Joel"

Joel was born a healthy baby. He reached all milestones within the normal range. I noticed changes in his behavior at about eighteen months. He talked less, had screaming tantrums at night and day. Joel no longer ate well and wouldn't stay dressed. The saddest part was Joel would bite himself and leave bruises on himself along with biting his parents.

Our local doctor said this was nothing to worry about, just a little delayed. Joel's dad finally agreed to formal testing when Joel turned five. School district's evaluation: Joel was functioning at eighteen months to two years, four months. Diagnosis: pervasive developmental delay. He was enrolled in a special education class, regional center program, and speech therapy. We supplemented with private speech classes and tutoring and seminars. Helping Joel was the focus of our entire lives, but none of it seemed to help. After all that Joel wasn't potty trained and barely talked. I heard about Dr. Goldberg from a parent at school. Joel started treatment with Dr. Goldberg at five and a half years old. Joel responded well to medication and dietary changes. Joel improved right away. Joel would respond when talked to, potty trained, took fewer naps during the day, and ate better. Joel then began to go through normal states of child development. He enjoyed being read to and enjoyed playing with kids a couple of years younger then himself.

We then tried regular school and speech therapy for the next two years. Joel was failing and lost confidence. Joel was set up to fail at school. Dr. Silton explained about stress and anxiety in Joel. She recommended we stop fighting with the school district, which doesn't know to how to help Joel. She then said to concentrate on getting Joel to relax and learn.

I found a retired teacher to tutor Joel plus speech at school. Joel calmed down and developed some confidence. He really enjoyed reading, math, and music. Next Joel was treated by an ENT specialist who helped with allergies and sinus problems. Joel's focus and attention and sleeping all night improved once again.

All this time Joel was seen by Dr. Goldberg every six to eight weeks, adjusting medications and diet. The last year that Joel required speech therapy was when he was ten years old. I would wait outside the classroom and once heard our special education director talking to Joel's speech pathologist. I heard her say, "I know this kid has this diagnosis, but I just don't see it." The speech pathologist replied, "I don't see it, either."

Joel is now twelve years old, and he is so much fun. He still has some challenges, but overall he's doing very well. I hope that better meds will be made available in the future to help with his strained immune system. He doesn't need any special education services or regional center services. Joel takes classes, plays sports, and plays with friends his own age.

Joel is doing so well that people can't believe he ever had the "A" label. People don't believe that their child can receive the same sort of results.

"Josiah"

Josiah was a very wanted and planned baby. For years his big sister asked for a sibling. Finally at seven years old her wish came true, and we welcomed baby Josiah. I remember looking at him thinking this is not a baby, but an old man. I gave birth to an old man! He was such a masculine baby, and just beautiful. Having another child, we can see he was developing typically. Josiah was a very connected and attached infant, and was gaining in all his milestones. At three months he knew my voice and would turn and search for me. He was so attached that I had to sneak out the back door to go to work. If he saw me leave, it was over! He cried like I broke his heart! I was his best girl. I still am!

He was a very happy baby. He looked at his big sister like she was the coolest thing in the world. As a baby the only illness he had was a bad case of thrush. It was very bad, though, and took a long time to go away. Next he had a bout of reflux that also persisted.

Josiah even spoke early, at nine months of age. He said his first words: "quack, quack." It wasn't just a one-time quack, either! Every time he saw a duck, he quacked his heart out! He even pointed. His next words were cars, go, ma, eat, juice, and soon at eleven months he said "cars go," and "good girl" to our family dog. His pediatrician even noted this was early for a two-word combination. I remember he would pet the dog sort of rough, yelling *"nice, nice,"* because we always said "be nice" to the dog. He was getting it. I always looked forward to coming home and being greated with "Hi!" as he ran into my arms. He played appropriately, was easy to take out, and was a big flirt with the ladies. We laughed at how he would totally ignore men and would reach out and grin at all the pretty ladies. Very social and a joy.

Soon at around fifteen months of age things started to change. He would cry over things that I didn't understand. There was no rhyme or reason. He became destructive and less verbal. Didn't want to walk, and would scream to be carried. Then he stopped talking. He had ten words and now had two left, "cars go." What happened to "Mom"? I never knew what he wanted. He got rigid, had to have things a certain way. He used to love going out to eat, this soon became torture. We would have to call ahead to the restaurant to order his meal, as he would rage if he had to wait. A few times a bus boy turned on the vacuum, and he went absolutely crazy. Even after the bus boy turned off the vacuum, he could not calm down. We had to leave immediately. Then he nearly stopped eating altogether. He would scream for milk all day. Why did he suddenly get calm when given milk, and erupt into a larger fit later? He no longer tolerated hats, haircuts, the merry-go-round, and no longer flirted with the ladies. He now would scream in the car, and hated outings. His bowel movements became so infrequent, and they affected his sleep. He would get strange fevers and seemed always sick. He no longer slept through the night. We often found him laughing hysterically in a dark room at 3:00 AM! This was scary!

On his developmental chart he was marked for the lowest amount of acceptable words. I took him several times, and was told not to worry. I remember when I was pregnant with his little sister, talking to the pediatrician about how I was concerned about him not understanding a baby was coming. She said just read to him "big brother" books, and he'll get it. By the time he was two and a half, his little sister was born, and he was shocked. He *never* understood a word of those big brother books. When I took her home, he looked at her and searched to see how he could take her apart. He searched for how her leg was attached. Like she was a doll, he then yanked hard trying to take her little leg off. He was very disappointed that she wasn't a doll. He just did not comprehend. By this time, I was finally told to worry. The wait-and-see approach lost us developmental time.

As he was evaluated, I kept saying to the psychologist, he can't be autistic, he's sick. I was told that whether he was sick or not, had no bearing on his diagnosis. My son did not play repetitively, and had great imaginative play. He loved touch, affection, and other than the "demon vacuum," he was fine with loud noises. During the evaluation, I remember them placing a cup, spoon, and a baby doll on the table. As they watched for inappropriate play, he places the baby in the cup, spins it, and says, "Weeeeeeeeee!" I watch the evaluator frown, and scribble something down. I said, "Wait, that is appropriate! We just got back from Disneyland and he loves the teacups!" She then erases her negative marks. Even though I spared him one negative point on her scorecard, I couldn't spare him the autism diagnosis. It was devastating. They were wrong. I felt firmly that he did not fit Kanner's definition of autism. Even then, I knew that this mislabel of autism would deny him a medical intervention. How could I get them to look deeper? I am just a mom.

As we immersed ourselves in the suggested therapies, I researched medical ways to treat his symptoms. First thing we tried was removing the milk from his diet. Josiah went through severe die-off from this that was completely scary. For nine days, he was gone. He stopped playing appropriately, stopped seeking affection, started lining things up, and was screaming in rage. I was scared we made it worse. He was doing things he never did before! Thankfully after ten days he started coming back. He stopped lining things up, and has never done it again. The best thing was he slept a bit better, screamed less, and gained thirty-three words in six weeks! We were on our way. He continued getting better when we added in antifungals and probiotics. My son's tongue was pink again. He was calmer and more focused. As we moved further in this popular autism protocol, we ran expensive labs and were told to remove all gluten as well as twenty-two other flagged foods. Strangely, when we did this, he got worse. He got strange fevers, the circles under his eyes worsened, he refused to eat, and he was miserable. I knew that we needed a new protocol.

I can remember when I found out about Dr. Goldberg, as I was up late one night Googling like a madwoman. I found his letter to Congress stating the most remarkable thing. He said it was "scientifically impossible for there to be a developmental epidemic." He further said that this epidemic was not autism, but a disease process. I cried as I read his words, as they made sense and provided hope. I called the next day, and was in his office six–eight weeks later. The first thing we did was change his diet. Dr. Goldberg's NIDS diet worked much better for him. Similar to GFCF, it was not hard to follow, but allowed more food. For my son, removing all those foods did him more harm than good. He was now milk free and whole grain free and feeling much better.

After receiving labs back indicating high titers of HHV6, we started antivirals. For Josiah, this was quite painful to start. My poor baby had massive headaches, stomachaches, night sweats, and excruciating leg spasms. I read on HHV6 adult boards that many experienced a sciatica-like pain in their legs and hands. I knew this was it, as he would suddenly scream and grab his foot and legs. He would curl up his little foot and scream for up to two hours. It was so hard to watch him go through. He would pinch his hands, as if they tingled, and whimper. In the middle of the night for the second week, he would wake constantly in a cold sweat. During this time I slept with him, and I was awakened one night to him slapping me while still asleep. He was completely asleep, and hitting and kicking me. As I protected myself with a pillow, I remember thinking, "It's okay, baby, fight that nasty virus!" For a while the virus seemed to stir up and grow, as his titers went up. Seeing this, Dr. Goldberg changed antivirals, and the virus dropped as well as all pains.

Josiah was the clearest we have ever seen. He was sleeping more, eating more, and he had gains in every direction. Because he was feeling better, we lost our terrible tantrums, and words were growing. He also began understanding language. He responded to his name again, and was here. I was floored when five months into the protocol, I asked him to clean up his mess and he did! One night, I said, "Okay, clear your plate," and he got up, scraped the food into the trash, put the plate in the sink, and clapped his hands and said, "*I did it!*" It was almost like he always wanted to listen, but couldn't. His words grew, from a vocabulary of 43 words to 135 words. He also learned to imitate.

Speech therapy began working better, as he would imitate sounds, then full words. Next were songs. It was beautiful to hear his little voice quietly singing, "Twinkle, twinkle little star." He even made up one short song of his own and marched through the house singing it. His play skills advanced developmentally, and he gained more imagination. He now loved to dress up and pretend to be different characters. His favorites were Buzz and Woody costumes. He would yell, "Yee haw!" and gallop around the house pretending to be Woody from *Toy Story*. His attention span grew, as he started to request stories to be read to him. This was amazing! He began to play with other children more, and his relationships with his sisters grew as well, especially with his older sister who was now eleven. She would say, "Mom, Josiah is so much fun now!" They were finally getting to know one another. As for his little sister, she was eighteen months and not as interesting, and he was still annoyed that he had to share his toys and his mommy with her.

The most amazing moment for me would sound strange to someone with typically developing children. I hold dear to my heart the moment that Josiah had a mini argument with me! It was *great*! I held in my smile, as he mocked me when I scolded him to eat his dinner. He yelled back, "Josiah, eat! Josiah, eat!" followed by roars of laughter. He then says, "No, no, no, no! You eat!" This continues for ten lovely minutes. I say lovely, because it was pure bliss to hear his voice so fluidly. He was the kid that had some words, but would *never* repeat a word when asked. Here he continues to mock me, yelling, "Not okay! You eat! No, no, no!" Then he wants to get down from his chair and says, "Down!" I say to him, "No down! First eat!" He thinks for a minute. And cleverly smiles and says, "Mom, hug!" He was manipulating me to get off his chair, and I was so proud! Awesome!

When he got back to school, five months after starting the protocol, the teachers and staff noted that he was more reachable and teachable. They were amazed. His teacher said that the lights were on, and his behaviors dropped significantly. He was more compliant, and he participated in class more. At home, he continued socially and making a friend. A girl, of course, as he is a little flirt again.

Josiah's road to recovery is a bumpy road, with ups and downs. It isn't an endless road, though, and I am grateful for a destination. After fifteen months on this protocol, I have noticed a clear correlation of how well he is doing and how high or low his HHV6 titers are. When his language drops and his behaviors rise, there is always a rise in titers or an ear infection brewing. My older daughter made a game to gauge his language. She got a tally counter, and from time to time start a competitive game of "How much can you get Josiah to talk?" A year ago this game would be impossible. We found that when his virus is down, and he is healthy we got a peak of 317 words in one day! This is amazing, as a year ago, it would be five words. We gauged when he was ill, and his virus was up and he was at a dragging thirty words a day. If this was genuine autism, how can we have these fluctuations? I feel this is further evidence that this is an illness.

Currently we are watching his titers drop again and seeing him come back to life. His relationship with his little sister has grown from tolerance to friendship. He now plays with her and loves her. It is so sweet to see him to ask for a Popsicle and reach for two, to give her one. He is growing to be a good big brother. If we can keep his ear infections from recurring, and his virus down, I feel he could fully recover in a couple of years. Keeping him healthy is proving trying, but at least he is with a doctor that believes in him.

He is not a lost boy anymore. He is here and is amazing!

Below are two journal entries from 2007, when he started to regress.

One is a schedule I was passing on to my mom, as she was about to care for the kids for the day.

The other is how the day *actually* proceeds. Although written in humor, it is all true.

Josiah's schedule; Written 2007

- Wakes by between 6:00 AM-9:00 AM (have juice out immediately)
- Playtime, diaper change
- Put out high chair one hour after he wakes, fix breakfast tray (pancakes w/butter syrup, strudel, peaches, etc.)

- If he doesn't eat put out snacks to graze (dry cereal, grapes, apples, banana, etc.)
- Playtime
- Time to unwind for nap. Put on less stimulating (classical baby) shows. Brush teeth. Try tickling him with toothbrush (I will show you how)
- Nap time starts between 10:00 AM–12 noon (nap only lasts for 2–2.5 hours).
- Wakes (have juice out immediately), diaper change
- Lunch is usually grazed. Leave out a corn dog, chicken fingers, dry cereal, or chips, and grapes or apples. If you can get him in a chair try peaches and yogurt.
- Playtime, graze, playtime, graze, playtime, graze (hopefully poop)
- Dinner is between 5:30–6:30 (put out chair fifteen minutes before)
- 1st, try thin pasta, or breaded chicken, 2nd give baby food veggies (in bowl he can dip spoon into), next clean up tray and give him drained peaches in a cup.
- You can choose to:
- 1. 5 min before he's done, have Soatikee (big sis) draw his bubble bath. Undress him in the kitchen and lead him to the bath, saying, "Oh, look at the bubbles!" Soatikee will wash his back and arms and watch him well, while you can recover the kitchen. (Hopefully he has pooped.)
- If you choose the above option, then if he ate enough, you can have a bottle warmed and ready by the bed, have his toothbrush ready, and a warm paper towel handy and dress him, brush his teeth, bottle him, wipe his teeth pacifier, and put him to bed. (Warning, he may have to poop after a warm bath, which means you will have to wait.)
- 2. Or you can delay his bath, just wipe his face/hands, have him play with Soatikee, (recover kitchen).
- Have him play (poop hopefully), and 1 hour later feed baby food at least one jar, have two handy though.

- Have Soatikee draw his bubble bath and start bathing him.
- While she is doing this get his stuff ready in the room. Warm toothbrush, warm paper towel, and warm bottle, and pacifier. Also have lotion, pj's, and towel ready. When he gets out, get him lotioned, dressed, brushed, bottled, burped, and put to bed.
- This is all subject to change and depends if he has pooped yet! He needs one to two good poops a day for an easier night.

Thank you for watching the rugrats for us. This means a lot to us.

Josiah's day, 2007

(Pay attention, there are tips in here that can get you through your day too!)

- He wakes up happy, continuing his thoughts on last night's conversation.
- topic: "Cars go!"
- Happiness quickly fades as he makes his way from the bedroom.
- His legs turn to jelly as he realizes he is no longer in bed, and he is quickly thrown into a bad mood for about an hour.
- Any quick movements are perceived as hostile toward him, so make your way through the morning cautiously.
- Offering juice too early is pretentious to him and unforgivable.
- Offering juice too late makes him think you're trying to dehydrate him and throws him into a panic.
- Better to have made the juice cup the night before and simply take out of the fridge and place in a central location.
- No, you cannot make the juice in the morning! If he sees you make juice, it will give him anxiety, and he will panic that you are going to pour juice forever and never give it to him!
- Breakfast is quickly denied after several tries. After he grazes a bit off his and your plate, he decides that this is wasting his time, and he has *a lot* to do this morning.
- And he is off! Lots of important things to do before his next tantrum.

- Got to: Pull cups out of the cupboard and drop them all over the house, empty the cat food by spilling all over kitchen and sliding on top of it belly first, take a few bites of cat food of course, check on the dog water ensuring freshness by sampling it, wake up all the pets with a "Nice" greeting, pull all the DVDs off the wall shelf, take out my Flintstones-type car and run over the dog, see if Mom is cleaning the cat food up right and "help" her by rolling on top of what she is sweeping up, the sliding glass door isn't sparkling; better lick it. Oh Mom is making the bed, better help her out by putting the sheets over my head and running into the walls, ah, she takes sheets away and makes the bed; time for medium-sized fit. Cardio exercise always makes him feel better, so he now runs around the house slamming all the doors. Quickly raises his heart rate by getting angry that the door he shut clicked shut, and he can't reopen.
- Now it is time for a large-size tantrum which involves rolling on the floor, crying at Mommy, and pushing her to sit down (as she is still cleaning up his mess) and make her cuddle him. He finds his pacifier on the couch and begins to self-soothe.
- Rubbing eyes show fatigue, but there is still some fight left! He is 21.9 months and is not going down yet!
- Time to play with sister and destroy her room. After she selfishly takes her favorite toy from his teeth, he begins a pretty good-sized meltdown. As he screams slamming doors looking for Mommy, he gets angered even more to find she is not where he left her. Where is she? As he cries looking for Mommy, he forgets why he was angry to begin with, and now is angry that she has moved from the spot he left her in. He soon finds her in the bathroom and quickly screams his way in. She washes her hands, scoops him up, and lays him down for nap. This is so offensive that she offers a nap without a bottle in her hand! She gives in and grabs a bottle and he is off to reenergize with a nap. He needs to, next will be lunchtime and more to do! It

will be time for an outing, more things to explore, put in his mouth, pee on, and he will need more energy to go, go, go!

"Jaxon"

I had a very hard time getting pregnant and staying pregnant (but I was oh so happy *being* pregnant, especially when I found out it was with twins!). I had my first contractions at nineteen weeks, when I was put on bed rest for a week and given a course of antibiotics for a suspected infection. At twenty-two weeks, I was in labor. I was admitted to our local hospital for one night and given magnesium sulfate via IV to see if it would stop the contractions. The next morning, I was transported by ambulance 1.5 hours from home and admitted to a hospital with a level IV NICU. I stayed there for twenty-eight days, contracting the whole time. My daughter was head down, engaged in the birth canal and I was dilated to 3 cm, so I was put in Trendelenburg position (head down, feet up), and told to stay on my left side as much as possible. I relied on my nurses for everything. My husband stayed by my side as much as possible the first week, my mother the second week, my brother in law the third week. The fourth week, friends stepped in to keep me company. By the twenty-eighth day, labor was unstoppable, and my beautiful babies were born at twenty-six weeks and two days gestation. Beautiful in our eyes, but in reality, they looked a bit like what I might describe as aliens. They weighed just two pounds each, which was quite large for twenty-six-week micropreemies.

We joke now that our daughter was a NICU troublemaker, but our son was let out early for good behavior. He needed very little oxygen support for being born so early, and he was considered a grower-feeder by the fourth week. It meant I could hold him anytime the NICU was open, and feed him and change his diapers and otherwise start bonding with him. He seemed to melt into me when I kangaroo'd him, where I held him skin-to-skin against my chest for long periods of time. We were still tethered to his incubator by wires and tubes that recorded his respirations and heartbeats, which I could watch on a monitor as they lulled me into a sense of security. When we brought him home three and a half weeks before his due date, he was, for all intents and purposes, a typical, healthy baby. Which was a miracle. They say

God only gives you what you can handle. His twin sister was released from the NICU after I begged and pleaded to take her home with a gavage feeding tube. I could not visit her in the NICU when I had my son to care for, and the challenge of trying to be in two places at once was more than I could bear. They both needed me equally, but NICU rules prohibited him from passing through the doors once he had been exposed to the outside world. She was experiencing intense reflux, so learning to take a bottle was proving a challenge, and her overscheduled day nurse did not have the time or patience to nurture our daughter the way she needed. She had had heart surgery when they were eight days old, then developed pneumonia and her lungs were, in the words of one of the neonatologists, "crap." She would take a couple of sips from a bottle, then pull away to take deep gulps of air. It made the reflux worse, and on top of that, the reflux made feeding painful.

We brought them home on a hot summer day. He had spent seventy-eight days in the NICU; she one hundred. I had lived in a wonderful Ronald McDonald House from the time I had been released from the hospital, after spending thirty-one days there myself, 1.5 hours from home and my husband and our beautiful, sweet dog. Nothing had felt better in my whole life than to walk back through my front door with both of my babies in my arms.

The first few weeks home were mostly a blur. Fortunately, we had the love of our families all around us, and nonstop visitors the first five weeks we were home from the hospital. Thank God, because I soon learned I could not put my daughter down for very long. She needed to be upright to help with her reflux and her breathing. Our first night home, she developed a very strange cry. Unbeknownst to me, a home health nurse appeared from nowhere (actually, she had been sent by the NICU to check in on us), which was quite a blessing because my daughter's oxygen levels were in the fifties. This started my all-consuming preoccupation with my daughter during their first two years of life. I don't remember very much about my son as an infant and a toddler, except that he was the easiest "dream baby," and I adored him. He slept a lot, and did not fuss much when he was awake, but he seemed to love cuddling, and he felt so good when I held him. He always made me feel as though everything in the world was just right. He had this funny habit of kicking his feet really, really hard until his socks were off, then he would settle back down and sleep for five or six hours at a time. When he was really fussy for some reason (reflux?), we would buckle him into his car seat or very early on he loved his swing and he would settle right down. We were visited weekly by the home health nurse. She would measure and weigh my babies, which was always very stressful, because my daughter was not gaining weight like she should have been. My son was growing just fine, but one day the nurse pointed out that he was not tracking an object she was moving back and forth. He also was not clasping his hands in front of him like most babies his age.

Their age was subjective for the first three years. There was their actual age (the time since their actual birth) and their adjusted age (the age they would be—3.5 months younger—if they had been born on their due date). Every time they were assessed, we were told they may/may not be delayed based on either of these "ages." I felt like they (we) were constantly under some kind of microscope.

At twelve months (actual), I noticed that he didn't play in the sandbox at the playground like his sister did. He preferred to pull himself up on the wheel of our jogger stroller and kind of rock back and forth. He was fascinated with wheels of all kinds, and would try to crawl after kids riding their bikes around the playground. I had to start watching him very carefully to make sure he didn't get his tiny little fingers stuck in any spokes or crushed under a rolling tire. At home, he played a funny game with himself that cracked us up! He had a "giggle ball" that made funny sounds as it rolled around. It was not perfectly round, either, so it didn't roll like a typical ball. He would bat at it and it would roll under the furniture, and he would laugh and chase it as fast as he could (not walking yet, it was kind of a commando-scramble), then get himself tangled in the legs of the furniture. He would seem to be getting frustrated, but then he would figure it out on his own, extricate himself, and start all over again. He also had a favorite baby wind chime toy, and he would bat at it for very long periods of time. I loved the pleasant tinkling sound it made, so it didn't bother me, until one day, I realized he didn't really play with their millions of toys like his twin sister did.

At ten months (actual), she had a favorite book of Noah's ark animals. She would point to every one of them and ask, "Dat?" and look to me until I answered. Her first word was at eleven months, "guck" (for duck). She *loves* anything to do with animals. He would spend all his time (when he wasn't sleeping, which he did for hours every day) chewing on a set of stainless-steel measuring spoons, chasing the "giggle ball," batting at the baby-chime, or dance-flying in the baby jumper. He could really get it going and then hold his feet up and fly through the air like Peter Pan!

I asked their OT if there could be a problem with him, right around the time they were fourteen months old. She said he was really too young to say with any certainty, but that he was being watched closely, and that she was encouraged because he responded really well when she had done any work with him to catch him up to his developmental milestones.

For example, when he should have been using his hands to grasp objects, he kept them fisted. The OT did some work with him, and in a matter of a couple of days (not sessions, but days) he was using his hands. She also got them to turn over on schedule and pull up and encouraged us to do floor-time exercises from three months forward.

At seventeen months (fourteen adjusted), his twin started walking. She was much smaller, but far more agile and—seemingly—stronger. One day, as she flew (I mean ran) around the house, I caught him watching her intently. I thought to myself, "He's going to start walking!" We had consulted with a PT, who had already done an evaluation and determined that he did have some muscle weakness (his hips seemed to give out when he tried to use their toy meant to help them walk, like the toddler version of a walker), and she had scheduled an appointment to work with him. The next day after watching his sister, he stood up in the middle of the room and walked across it, holding on to nothing! He never received PT to help with walking. He didn't need or receive PT until he started preschool, and he received adaptive PE.

That's our boy. He amazes us all the time. He has always responded really well to most of the therapies and interventions. He has been a patient of Dr. Goldberg for the last 4.5 years. I really don't know where he would be if it weren't for the NIDS protocol and Dr. G. But I'm getting ahead of myself. Let me go back to when he was a toddler and started showing signs of illness.

My son was always very sweet and affectionate with us. He ran to the front door when my husband came home from work, and allowed me to cuddle with him at naptime and bedtime. He loved singing songs like "Itsy Bitsy Spider," holding his little hand to mine so we could do the motions together, even though he used no words to communicate with us. His twin and I always seemed to know exactly what he needed. He never had tantrums or cried much. He always "went with the flow" and he could—and did—fall asleep anywhere. He has always made up lost sleep. I was worried about his lack of words, but not too much. The ST, who was working with my daughter for ongoing feeding challenges (which turned out to be due to an intolerance to corn), kept an eye on him.

At eighteen months (actual), both of my babies received a flu shot, then came down with rotovirus a few days later. Looking back, I believe this was his "tipping point." He was sick from that point forward. He started getting rashes around his mouth and on his body when he ate certain foods that had never been a problem before. He started getting ear infections and had some respiratory infections (lower and upper), and he had strep a few times. He had an ear infection or fluid in his ears from eighteen months to four and a half years old, and three sets of ear tubes. His tonsils were very large and red until he was seven. His adenoids were removed when he was four, but it didn't help. When he got sick, it would last for months. He had thick, green mucous coming out of his nose for at least a year. When he was three and a few months, he started drooling. Three-year-olds don't just start drooling. I took him to the dentist and the pediatrician, but neither had an explanation.

I am not against vaccinations, but I think they need to be given a lot more intelligently than they were given to my son. He was given five vaccinations in the NICU, one month before his due date when he weighed four pounds. Two months later, he was given four more in one day. All of his vaccinations were given on schedule, often when he was sick. At fourteen months (actual), he was being unsuccessfully introduced to cow's milk and given the MMR at the same time.

The illnesses help explain his development (his developmental delays, I should say). When my babies were two, I started taking them to a pre-preschool. It was really fun to go there one day a week, especially since we lived in a remote area, they were considered medically fragile (my daughter, especially) and we didn't have many options for socializing. He would get so excited when we went there, and he would zing from one toy to another. The director commented once to me, in a not very kind or informative way, "At this age, he *should* be able to sit in circle time." Circle time was completely new to me. My daughter had no problem sitting on my lap for fifteen to twenty minutes, singing the songs with the other toddlers and listening to a story. As a toddler he was a huge fan of Winnie the Pooh and had all the characters. He has always loved Disneyland. He also loved *Cars* and loved to play with cars like most toddlers. So when we were at the school, I thought he was just very excited to be in a new environment and wanted to experience as much of it as possible. We tried "Mommy & Me" music, but the instructor asked us not to come back. The class was held in her home (which was not toddler-proofed) and she feared for his safety. He refused to participate and instead ran from one thing in her home to another while I tried to provide his twin sister with an enriching experience.

At two years, ten months, I tried to enroll him in a Montessori preschool. My thinking was that he just needed regular exposure to an environment away from our home. He was so clearly different in that environment; it was a huge eye-opener for me. He was definitely in his own world at the preschool, and did not notice the other children or one of the two directors (he latched on to the blond director, no problem, but wanted/needed nothing to do with anyone else). Of concern at this time was the fact that he did not point at things, did not have good eye contact, and tended to go off by himself. A developmental psychologist did a full evaluation, observing my son in the preschool, our home, and his office. He also interviewed my husband and me extensively. He told us he was so sorry, but that he was going to give him a diagnosis of autism spectrum disorder. He told us he wasn't 100 percent sure as he didn't fit the diagnosis perfectly, but he didn't fit other diagnoses, either. My son, no matter what his diagnosis was, needed help, and he needed it right away. He was delayed in speech, motor, and social skills. The psychologist gave him the diagnosis so my son could receive the services he needed, and he felt that someday, we would come back to him and the diagnosis would no longer fit. We were devastated and numb, but it didn't take me long to start trying to figure out what to do to help him.

One of the first things I did was attend a TACA parent meeting. The guest speaker that first night had written a book about the journey she had been on with her son. Dr. Goldberg was one of the main characters. I bought her book that night and finished reading it before I went to sleep. The next day, I contacted Dr. Goldberg's office to get an intake packet. I returned the completed packet within a week. It was at least one inch thick with my very young son's history. We got our first appointment for approximately three months later. It was while waiting for this appointment that my now three-year-old son started drooling.

We also started the GFCF diet during the wait. I also removed soy and preservatives. I saw some immediate changes in his behavior. He was less hyper, for one. We were desperate to get his twin sister to grow and gain weight during this time, and I had even resorted to Pop-Tarts as a snack at the playground. I noticed that within a few minutes after eating them, he was clobbering her on the head as he rode behind her in our double stroller. That's when I started limiting sugar and food dyes.

At our first appointment with Dr. G., I was so impressed because he had read and studied my son's history. His chart was full of yellow sticky notes, and Dr. G. went through it with me and asked questions for clarification. At the end of the three-hour visit, he told me my son does not have autism, and that he could help him. He ran blood work, and we headed home. I felt like we were in good hands and my son would be well cared for. My mom was at the visit, as well. She has worked for medical researchers for years, and she knew a lot of what Dr. G. told us about retroviruses and how my son became so sick, and what could and would be done to help him. This really "fit" for me, since my son also has a diagnosis of cerebral palsy. I had read that thirty-some percent of preemies that developed CP developed it due to exposure to a herpes-related virus around the time of their birth, and not due to a hypoxic event. My son was given five vaccinations at one time in the NICU, one month before his due date and another four vaccinations at one time two months later. I believe these vaccinations helped compromise his already-immature immune system. If the vaccinations themselves didn't contain the viruses (which they likely did), then his immune system was unable to defend him against exposure while he was assimilating them.

Not long afterward, another mom recommended a local osteopath who also had cerebral palsy. I took my son to him for a consultation. Without discussing with him Dr. G. or the protocol, he told me, too, that my son did not have autism and that he could become well.

The NIDS protocol has included antivirals (Famvir, Valtrex, Zovirax), antifungals (Diflucan, Nizoral), low doses of a SSRI (by far the scariest part for me to give my son, until I saw how they helped his focus and attention), anti-inflammatory diet (difficult at times until we accustomed to it, but so essential), probiotics, antihistamines, Tenex (for impulsivity), DHA-EPA, a good multivitamin, and iron. We also had to use mineral oil for years for chronic constipation, which is now resolved.

His therapies have included floor time, ABA, speech, occupational therapy, physical therapy and music therapy, plus Brain Highways and, of course, the NIDS protocol. He wore braces on his legs because he walked on his toes (he even walked with his toes curled under!).

Fast-forward to today. My son is eight and in second grade. He has been fully included in a typical classroom since kindergarten. He has missed one day for illness this year. That's almost a miracle. In preschool he missed weeks' worth of school for illness. In kindergarten, he missed approximately twenty days. Last year, it was less than ten. He has several friends at school, and he is well liked by his peers and the staff. His teachers love him. He is at or above academic level in almost every area. He is regulated most of the time, and he has even learned how to help regulate himself. His language is still somewhat delayed, but he is becoming conversational and is quite witty and has a great sense of humor. During the summer between second and third grades, he will spend several hours working with FastForward to help his language comprehension develop and hopefully catch him up developmentally 100 percent. He loves being on the go, camping with his dad and Adventure Guides, roller coasters, riding bikes, going to the beach and Boogie Boarding, and playing with his twin sister and his friends at school, swimming, and taking pictures with his camera. He is a whiz on the computer, too. He is not 100 percent recovered yet, but I do foresee full recovery, and he now appears pretty typical, at least in most situations. I know he will drive a car, attend college, have a career, live independently, and, if he wants, have a family of his own. He will be a productive member of society and contribute instead of needing a lifetime of care. We were blessed with early intervention, with people who knew what they were doing, and who really cared about my son, and I am thankful for people like Dr. Goldberg, who is willing to try new protocols and is stretching out to find the answers for these kids who are so very special. Our son is an amazing gift and is a delight to everyone who knows him. This journey has been physically, emotionally, and financially exhausting, but also has enriched and touched our family, our school district, our friends, and the therapists and medical community in so many wonderful ways. Our son is full of surprises for us all, and he is one of the happiest people I know. I feel honored I was chosen to be his mom.

"Simon"

"The recital is coming," says Simon's guitar teacher. "Do you want to play 'Ode to Joy'? It is next Saturday."

I almost opened my mouth to reply, but decided to let my son to handle the conversation. "Sure," he said, "I can make up my art lesson on Wednesday instead of Saturday, Mom."

It was quiet in the car on our way home. Simon was reading his book, and I was thinking. "Ode to Joy." Sure. Why not? How symbolic. My memory brought me back to my childhood. I was about Simon's age when we started learning about Beethoven in my music school. It was a while ago in Russia. I remember my teacher's remark about Ninth Symphony, the beginning. "That's how destiny knocks on your door. Ta-da-da-da . . ."

Destiny knocked to our door as to many other doors when Simon was less then three years old. Like many other parents, we've realized that he is developmentally delayed, but when Simon's preschool teacher called me for a talk, we've realized that things are getting serious.

Simon got his diagnosis pretty fast. First it was PDD-NOS, which they quickly changed to autism. By the time the University of Minnesota clinic gave his report, we already knew the diagnosis. After initial shock and anger we started to do our research. We knew we didn't have time for grief. After hours of web searching and spending a good sum of money on books, we've decided to move quickly, just start with something, anything that is available to help our son.

It was easier said than done. We've both had very demanding jobs and older child to take care of. The school district was not much help. They provided only ten hours a week of special education, and the curriculum was not very impressive. Mostly they tried to teach us how to accept Simon's condition. "Just love him," his teachers said. And there were plenty of parents who did just that. I attended a parent support group meeting only once and left after one mom with two autistic kids said, "I am even happy they are autistic!" I was not happy at all.

I have a master's degree in biology, and my husband is physicist. Being a biologist helped me a lot. I quickly realized that we had to find medical treatments for Simon's condition, not just behavioral ones. I put him on the GFCF diet at once. It helped a lot. We've had initial success with DAN treatment, but things looked very uncertain and complicated.

Finding a good program for Simon looked almost impossible. All home agencies were booked, and besides, we did not have any funds to pay for it. We were stuck with the school district, with our DAN doctor and me, personally, with a very unhappy manager in my lab.

I read about NIDS at the very beginning of my endless search for information. It made lots of sense to me. I even tried to find someone in Minnesota to help me to implement the protocol. I have family in

California and we visit often, but to go to Los Angeles just to see a doctor? Anyway, I joined the NIDS Yahoo group and started to read e-mails.

I cannot recall the moment I decided to make an appointment. I think it was after a conversation with one Minnesota mom whose son was among the first of Dr.Goldberg patients helped us to make our mind.

The waiting list was long (six months) but someone canceled. I immediately took the spot. We came to California just before Simon's third birthday. Around the same time the first center-based ABA agency opened in Minnesota, and our insurance paid for treatment. It was almost a miracle. Simon went to this place from 8:30 till 5:30 every day like to preschool.

Simon now is eleven. He "graduated" from his therapy just before kindergarten and he is another "success story" for the agency's owner. They provided very valuable service. We still get phone calls from new clients and gladly give references.

On our late visit to Dr. Goldberg's office we saw Simon's file. It was huge and probably is going to be bigger. We are not going to "graduate" from it easily. I cannot tell my son when he can stop to take his medication or when he can try other types of food. I cannot promise him that we are not going to do NeuroSPECT anymore. And he cannot stop coming to the hospital for blood drawing every six weeks.

People who did not know about Simon's condition cannot even suspect that something is wrong with him. His teachers at school know, though he does not get any special services. His art teacher does not know. Neither do his swim team coaches or his guitar teacher.

Our life is not going in the direction we planned so long ago. We are constantly compromising and planning ahead. Everything that Simon does analyzed carefully. We constantly ask ourselves, is he normal? Does he behave as a typical child? What do other kids think about him?

Our road is still bumpy. We constantly fight allergies, virus, and low white blood cell count. Simon looks and behaves much better than his monthly blood work does. His latest NeuroSPECT is not as good as we had hoped. There is still a lot to be done.

I have only one piece of advice to other parents: Do not be afraid to change your life. Do not be afraid to go to another state to get the best care. Do not be afraid of making your child cry when the nurse has to draw his blood. Do not be afraid to rearrange your life and house. We all have our life planned to a certain extent and we do not like to accept changes.

So, did we successfully come to "Ode to Joy"? Hopefully for us it will end better than for Beethoven. For him "Ode to Joy" was the end. I believe, for us it is just a beginning.

"Kaylie"

Our little girl was diagnosed with PDD at two and a half. Like other parents, we were not given a whole lot of hope. They told us there was no "cure," it was a "developmental disorder", and that she would never be like other children. Our best option would be to get her into the best behavioral program we could find. That was it. They did no medical workup whatsoever. These were top Boston doctors in top Boston hospitals. When I asked about special diets or immune system problems or anything that may have been metabolical or biological, they dismissed every bit of it. Pretty soon we dismissed them. We tried a DAN doctor but still didn't get the answers we were seeking. Other parents around the web were raving about Dr. Goldberg. After poring over his website, I knew he was the one for our Kaylie. His science made a lot of sense. "Are you crazy?" was my husband's first reaction. "He is in California. We are in Massachusetts. He sounds great, but it's just not possible." Then I learned that Dr. Goldberg came to the East Coast a couple times a year. So when Kaylie was in kindergarten and six years old, she met Dr. Goldberg for the first time.

Kaylie was progressing nicely with her behavioral/educational component before she started with Dr. Goldberg. As she started the medications, we noticed her progress markedly sped up. It was easier for her to focus and remain calm. The lingering problem behaviors all went away and she seemed happier. She went on to regular first grade on her own and did great. By the end of grade 1, she no longer qualified for any special education services and was considered a "typical" child. I remember crying a lot that year. It is hard to explain the overwhelming appreciation and joy a parent of a special needs child feels when they see their child accomplish something that once seemed impossible. We of course still saw little things that needed work. And her blood work still showed that there were problems. Over the years, her blood work slowly improved, and Kaylie socially matured.

Today Kay is fourteen and is about to graduate from eighth grade. She is an honor student who is super excited about the big eighth grade dinner dance that's coming up. She spends a good deal of time either listening to her iPod, texting on her cell phone, or talking to friends on the computer. I guess you could say she is a typical teen. She understands what happened to her and that her body was sick. She hates the "A" word; in fact she leaves the room if it comes on TV. She's such a good girl. Life has not been easy for her, but she doesn't complain. Even when she has to endure a painful shot, she doesn't flinch. When she knows I will be talking to Dr. G, she sometimes asks when he is going to get the medicine that lets her eat pizza and "normal" food. I guess that would be her one complaint. She wants to eat the junk she sees her pals eating.

If not for Dr. Goldberg, Kaylie would not be where she is today. What if we had listened to the Boston specialists? They didn't draw blood. They didn't look at her brain. How much damage would have been done to my daughter's brain and body by now if we had done what the Boston doctors recommended? I doubt she would be taking honors algebra right now. It is scary and sad. Those Boston waiting rooms were full of kids just like Kaylie. Not all parents question doctors. How many of those kids could have been with my daughter right now if their parents had been given the right information and the right treatment? We are so appreciative for all Dr. Goldberg has done for Kaylie and how hard he has worked for our kids. We only hope that soon there will be a lot more support for NIDS. In a couple of weeks, we will be attending Kaylie's eighth grade graduation. We are so proud of Kaylie for all she has overcome, and full of tremendous gratitude for Dr. Goldberg, for giving Kaylie the means to a healthy, normal life. She is on her way to high school and then off to fulfill wherever her dreams take her. She has done all they said could never be done.

"Noah"

"He's going to be an early talker," Robyn announced to her husband, Greg, while playing with their four-and-a-half-month-old son, Noah. The baby responded with soft coos and gurgling sounds. His mouth moved as if words were scrambling to get out. Noah's older brother, Joshua, was never much of a babbler, his mother recalled. He was a quiet, happy child, but he wasn't prone to labeling objects or uttering single words. When Joshua began to talk at about thirteen months, he did so in complete, oftentimes grammatically correct sentences.

Excited, the mother of two sons was anxious to hear Noah begin to attach meaning to the world around him through language. At a year, he was still babbling, but there was no progression toward meaningful language. Robyn and Greg voiced their concern to Noah's pediatrician but were assured there was nothing wrong with their baby boy.

Then, things got worse. Noah stopped babbling and began to avoid eye contact. He didn't respond to his name and rarely smiled. Noah cried a lot, ran unexplained high fevers, and developed a full body rash that doctors couldn't explain. His sleep was restless, and he seemed content to stay in his crib and stare at the ceiling. At age thirteen months, Noah crawled but refused to walk. Dismayed by the unexpected turn of events, Robyn and Greg began to press their pediatrician for answers.

"We suspected something was wrong," Robyn said. "We just didn't know what."

The doctor recommended x-rays to ensure Noah's legs physically were fine. The x-rays were negative; there was no medical reason to explain why he wasn't walking. At the time, Robyn was pregnant with their third child, Elijah. Soon after his birth, they switched insurance plans and started seeing a new pediatrician. Finally at the age of twenty two months, Noah began to walk, but he still had no words. Again, Robyn and Greg voiced their concerns over their son's developmental delays at his annual checkup. The new pediatrician encouraged the couple to give him some more time.

"The doctor thought that we were probably comparing Noah to Joshua, because he was highly verbal and reading by the time he was three years old," said Greg.

Unsatisfied, the parents insisted on referrals to any specialists who might help.

"We dragged him to an audiologist to check his hearing and then to a speech pathologist to assess his preverbal skills and general development," Robyn said. "She was the first person to actually suggest there was something wrong with him."

With a referral to a psychologist in hand, Robyn left the clinic feeling like someone finally was listening. Two weeks later, Robyn and Greg had their answer. At the age of two and a half, their precious baby boy was diagnosed with autism, or what was labeled as autism.

The same day Noah was diagnosed, Robyn left her three children with her sister and attended a support group meeting in Los Angeles.

"One mother asked me how I could be so calm. Her son had been diagnosed a couple of months ago, and she still felt paralyzed," Robyn said. "I told her that now our enemy had a name, and it was our job as Noah's parents to fight for him."

After months of research and referrals, the family embarked on a journey, which included ABA, speech therapy, vitamins, and enzymes. Although Noah made some progress, he was still having tantrums, severe hyperactivity, and difficulty with fine motor skills. He would speak one-to-two word sentences, but only when he desperately wanted something.

"It seemed that with every step forward, he would take two steps back," noted his father. "It was very frustrating."

When Noah was five years old, he started having seizures. Joshua had been diagnosed the year before with a seizure disorder. Soon after that, Noah developed another neurological condition called cyclical vomiting syndrome (CVS) and excruciating migraines. For nearly two years, Noah would throw up for several days out of each month, with migraines before and after each episode. There is no effective treatment for CVS except antinausea drugs, which rarely helped. Imitrex nasal spray eased the pain of the migraines.

"It was devastating to watch Noah go through this month after month, with no end in sight. We were virtual shut-ins during these episodes," Robyn said. "It was particularly hard on Joshua and Elijah."

Desperate, Robyn and Greg made the decision to take Noah off all vitamins and supplements. Robyn painstakingly searched the Internet for answers and happened upon the website of Dr. Michael Goldberg.

"When I read the description of neuroimmune dysfunction syndrome and what it does to the brain, I realized that it perfectly described my son," said Robyn.

NIDS occurs from a dysregulated immune system. The malfunction can be triggered by a virus, stress in utero or after the baby is born, illness, or trauma.

After reviewing the website, Greg, a skeptic by nature, enthusiastically agreed to a visit with Dr. Goldberg. Seven-year-old Noah had his first appointment in January of 2008. His lab tests indicated immune dysfunction. Four months into the protocol, the CVS completely stopped. The migraines continued, but with less frequency and intensity. Now, after two years, he is steadily progressing in school. Noah is learning to read and loves to draw. He seeks out his brothers to play a game of Wii or jump on the trampoline. Noah's speech has improved markedly. He speaks in five-to-seven word sentences. He asks questions and provides answers, all the while maintaining eye contact.

"We have a long way to go, but he is finally fully participating in the journey," said his proud father. "Our steps are consistently forward now."

Right before Noah began his treatment, Robyn and Greg began to notice issues with Joshua and Elijah. Joshua's eczema was out of control, and despite being extraordinarily bright, he was having difficulty in school. Unfortunately, he had Asperger's syndrome, a high-functioning form of autism where the child is highly verbal but socially impaired. Elijah, now five years old, was suffering from night terrors, ADHD, and extremely defiant behavior.

"He would wake up in the morning with dark purple circles under his eyes, and despite ten hours of sleep, he was exhausted," said Robyn.

On one of the family's many trips to the neurologist for Joshua and Noah, the doctor observed Elijah's erratic and unpredictable behavior and told Robyn that he probably would be seeing him as a patient sooner or later.

"I really thought we were heading for a diagnosis of ADHD or worse, bipolar disorder," said Robyn. "That thought terrified me."

First Joshua and then Elijah began to see Dr. Goldberg. Their lab work was eerily similar to Noah's. After about six months of treatment, Robyn and Greg began to see remarkable improvements in both boys. Their immune systems began to normalize, and with that came improvements in behavior, cognition, and overall health. Joshua recently made the principal's list, and Elijah is excelling in first grade. Both Joshua and Noah have been weaned off seizure medication and have not had a seizure in almost a year.

"Our children are sick and in pain. It's no wonder they have tantrums, difficulty learning, and become withdrawn," Greg said. "Although some of their symptoms mirror autism, this is not true autism."

Robyn and Greg believe, as do others whose children have seen progress on the NIDS protocol, that this disorder is neither psychiatric nor developmental in nature. It is NIDS—a medical illness that is robbing many children of their strength, their health and their future.

"This crisis is stealing an entire generation," said Robyn. "But with Dr. Goldberg's help, we are determined that our children will not be among them."

APPENDIX C

○ ○ ○ ◉ ○ ○ ○

PATIENT SCREENING/DATA QUESTIONNAIRE FOR AUTISM/PDD/ADHD USED AT DR. GOLDBERG'S PRACTICE

(Review fully—correlate issues with other workups and past evaluations)

Name: Last:_____ First:_____ ID#_____
DOB:_____ Age (at time of "intake" evaluation) _____ Sex:__
Initial Visit _____month _____day _____year _____

Entering Diagnosis: _____
Date: Dx: Physician/Psychologist Specialty
1. _____
2. _____
3. _____
4. _____

Maternal Hx:/PMH:

Pregnancy:

Problems during pregnancy_____
Gestation Term:_____ Premature:_____ wks _____ months
Ultrasound: Y___ N___ #_____
Delivery: Vaginal_____ C-Section_____ Normal_____ Apgars: 1)__ 5)__
Problems _____
_____
_____

Neonatal hx: Normal _____Abnormal_____
Problems: _____
_____
Other: _____
_____

History of:

Maternal fever: _____
Maternal bleeding: _____
Perinatal or Neonatal asphyxia:_____

Neonatal infection: _____

Maternal miscarriages: _____

Abortions: _____

Other: _____

_____

Maternal Medication:_____Which Trimester:_____

Drug Exposure: Y___ N___ Alcohol: Y___ N___ Explain: _____

_____

Family History:

_____

_____

_____

Siblings:	**B.D.**	**Order/Rank:**
1)		
2)		
3)		
4)		

Learning Disorder Y_____N_____

Describe: _____

Psychological Disorder Y_____N_____

Describe: _____

Autoimmune Disease Y_____N_____

Describe: _____

Rheumatoid Y___N___

Describe: _____

Lupus Y___N___

Describe: _____

Migraines/Allergies Y___N___

Describe: _____

Other _____

_____

Genetic Disorder Y___N____ Describe: _____

Cholesterol Abnormalities Y___N____ Describe: _____

Dementia: Y_____ N_____

Describe: _____

Psychiatric Disorder: Y_____ N_____

Describe: _____

Other: _____

_____

Developmental Hx:

Normal Developmental milestones till_____ months old

Sat-up_____ months. Walked_____ months

Babbling_____ months _____

Talked: N/A___ 4–6 words_____ 2–word sentences_____

any words_____

Descriptive use of words Y_____ N_____ When_____

Denver Developmental: _____

Vineland: _____

WISC-R: _____

CARS: _____

Echolasia Y_____ N_____ Comment _____

Self-Stemming: Y_____ N_____ Comment _____

Eye Contact: Poor_____ Good_____ Variable_____

Describe: _____

Other Developmental Difficulties: Y___ N___

Describe: _____

Sensory processing difficulty Y___ N___ **Onset:** _____

Describe: _____

Vestibular Dysfunction Y___ N___ **Onset:** _____

Describe: _____

Auditory Processing difficulty Y___ N___ **Onset:** _____

Describe: _____

Visual skill difficulty Y___ N___ **Onset:** _____

Describe: _____

Organization skill difficulty Y___ N___ **Onset:** _____

Describe: _____

Other strengths or weaknesses _____

_____

_____

Other: _____

_____

PMH:

Chicken pox: Y___ N___ Age:_____ Vaccine:_____

Frequent ear infections Y____ N_____ #_____

Bedwetting Y ___ N ___after the age of 5_____

Hx; of Allergies Y____ N____

Food: _____

_____

Asthma: Y___ N___ **Onset**_____ Active/Inactive

Hay Fever: Y___ N___ **Onset**_____ Active/Inactive

Eczema: Y___ N___ **Onset**_____ Active/Inactive

Migraines: Y___ N___ **Onset**_____ Active/Inactive

Medication: Y____ N____ Which_____

Hx of IBS_____ Constipation_____ Diarrhea_____

Seizures: Y___ N___ **Onset**_____ Type:_____

Describe _____

Other: _____

Hospitalizations: _____

_____

Other: _____

_____

Immunizations:

MMR Dates:_____ Reaction Y___ N___
Describe: _____
DPT Reaction Y___ N___ Not Given _____
Describe: _____

Psychosocial:

Behavioral Issues: Y___ N___ **Onset:**_____
Describe: _____
Affection: Y___ N___ Comment _____
Temper Tantrums Y___ N___ **Onset:**_____
Describe: _____
Fidgety/Hyperactive Y___ N___ **Onset:**_____
Describe: _____
Can't concentrate/easily distractible Y___ N___ **Onset:**_____
Describe: _____
Family Conflicts Y___ N___ Onset:_____
Describe: _____
Sleep Difficulties: Y___ N___ **Onset:**_____
Describe: _____
(i.e., Falling asleep_____ Frequent Waking_____ Tired in AM___)
Obsessive/Compulsive Tendencies: Y___ N___ **Onset:**_____
Describe: _____
Frustrated: Y___ N___ Describe:_____

_____

Activity Level: Hyper___ Normal____ Decreased/Lethargic_____
Variable_____ Describe:_____
Staring Spells: Y___ N___ **Onset:**_____
occasional_____ frequent_____ brief_____ prolonged_____
Desribe: _____
"Tuned-out" Y___ N___ **Onset:**_____

Describe: _____

Food Cravings: Y___ N___

Describe: _____

_____

Other: _____

_____

Autistic/PDD Profiles:

"Normal" till _____months _____year Describe _____

_____

Meet *DSMIII/IV* criteria for Autistic Disorder Y___ N___

PDD Disorder Y___ N____

Impairment in social interaction:

Impairment with nonverbal behaviors: Y___ N___ **Onset:**_____

Describe: _____

Failure to develop peer relationships: Y___ N___ **Onset:**_____

Describe: _____

Lack of sharing interests etc: Y___ N___ Onset:_____

Describe: _____

Lack of social or emotional reciprocity: Y___ N___ **Onset:**_____

Describe: _____

Impairments in communication:

Impairment to sustain or initiate speech: Y___ N___ **Onset:**_____

Describe:_____

Stereotyped or repetitive speech: Y___ N___ **Onset:**_____

Describe:_____

Lack of varied or spontaneous play: Y___ N___ **Onset:**_____

Describe:_____

Repetitive and sterotyped patterns of behavior, interests, and activities:

Inflexible adherence to rituals: Y___ N___ **Onset:**_____

Describe:_____

Repetitive motor mannerisms: Y___ N___ **Onset:**_____
Describe: _____
Persistent preoccupation with parts of objects Y___ N___ **Onset:**_____
Describe: _____

Physical Exam:

Dysmorphic Features: Y___ N___ Describe: _____
_____

Muscle Tone: Normal_____ Decreased_____ Increased_____
Neurologic Exam: Normal_____ Abnormal_____ Date:_____
Describe: _____
_____

Coordination: Normal_____ Abnormal____ Date:_____
Describe: _____
_____

Handedness: Right:_____ Left:_____ Ambidextrous_____
Cerebellar: Normal_____ Abnormal_____ Date:_____
Describe: _____
_____

Motor: Fine: Normal_____ Abnormal_____ Date:_____
Describe: _____
_____

Gross: Normal_____ Abnormal_____ Date:_____
Describe: _____
_____

Other: _____
_____

Past Lab:

Metabolic Screen:

Urine Amino Acids Normal____ Abnormal_____
Describe_____

Plasma Amino Acids Normal_____ Abnormal_____
Describe_____

Organic Acids Normal_____ Abnormal_____
Describe_____

Other _____

Chromosones: Normal: _____ Abnormal: _____ Date:_____
 Fragile X: Y_____ N_____ Type: _____
EEG: Y_____ N_____ Normal_____ Abnormal_____ Date:_____
Describe_____
_____
_____

NeuroSPECT: Y_____ N_____ Normal _____ Abnormal _____
Date_____
Location: HGA/UCLA _____ Other _____
Result _____
_____

MRI: Y_____ N_____ Normal_____ Abnormal_____ Date:_____
Describe_____
_____

Lead level: Normal_____ Abnormal_____ Describe _____
CBC: Normal_____ Abnormal_____ Describe _____

Chem Panel: Normal_____ Abnormal_____ Describe_____
Other:
_____
_____

GLOSSARY

ANA: Antinuclear antibody, an unusual antibody directed against structures within the nucleus of the cell. ANAs are found in patients whose immune system is predisposed to cause inflammation against their own body tissues. Antibodies that are directed against one's own tissues are referred to as autoantibodies. ANAs indicate the possible presence of autoimmunity.

ASD: Autism spectrum disorders (ASD), also called autism spectrum conditions (ASC) or the autism spectrum, with the word autistic sometimes replacing autism, are a spectrum of psychological conditions characterized by widespread abnormalities of social interactions and communication, as well as severely restricted interests and highly repetitive behavior.

atrophy: Atrophy is a general physiological process of reabsorption and breakdown of tissues, involving apoptosis on a cellular level. When it occurs as a result of disease or loss of trophic support due to other disease, it is termed pathological atrophy, although it can be a part of normal body development and homeostasis as well.

autoimmunity: The propensity for the immune system to work against its own body is referred to as autoimmunity.

bacteriocidal: An agent that destroys bacteria.

bacteriostatic: An agent, such as a chemical or biological material, that inhibits bacterial growth.

basal ganglia: The thalamus together with other closely related masses of gray matter, situated near the base of the brain.

brain stem: The portion of the brain, consisting of the medulla oblongata, pons Varolii, and midbrain, that connects the spinal cord to the forebrain and cerebrum.

brain tubulins: Tubulin is one of several members of a small family of globular proteins.

calcarine: Pertaining to, or situated near, the calcar of the brain.

CAT: Computed tomography (CT) or computed axial tomography (CAT) scanning uses a series of X-rays of the head taken from many different directions. Typically used for quickly viewing brain injuries, CT scanning uses a computer program that performs a numerical integral calculation on the measured X-ray series to estimate how much of an X-ray beam is absorbed in a small volume of the brain. Typically the information is presented as cross sections of the brain. In approximation, the more dense a material is, the whiter a volume of it will appear on the scan (just as in the more familiar "flat" X-rays). Rhodes Adair (of Harvard Medical School) is working on a new, more efficient version of the traditional CT scan. CT scans are primarily used for evaluating swelling from tissue damage in the brain and in assessment of ventricle size. Modern CT scanning can provide reasonably good images in a matter of minutes.

cerebellum: A region of the brain that plays an important role in the integration of sensory perception and motor control.

CFIDS: Chronic fatigue and immune dysfunction syndrome.

CFS: A condition characterized by disabling fatigue, accompanied by a constellation of symptoms, including muscle pain, multijoint pain without swelling, painful cervical or axillary adenopathy, sore throat, headache, impaired memory or concentration, unrefreshing sleep, and postexertional malaise. This diagnosis requires that a patient have four or more symptoms concurrently that persist for six or more months. The diagnosis is one of exclusion. Also called immune dysfunction syndrome.

cortical layers: Are composed of six somewhat distinct layers; each layer is identified by the nerve cell type and the destination of these nerve cell's axons (within the brain). The human cortex is a roughly 2.4 mm-thick sheet of neuronal cell bodies.

cytokines: Chemicals made by the cells that act on other cells to stimulate or inhibit their function.

delayed hypersensitivity: A cell-mediated response that occurs in immune people peaking at twenty-four to forty-eight hours after challenge with the same antigen used in an initial challenge. The interaction of T-helper 1 (Th-1) lymphocytes with MHC class II positive antigen-presenting cells initiates the response. This interaction induces the Th-1s and macrophages at the site to secrete cytokines, which are the major factors in the reaction. Called tuberculin-type hypersensitivity. Synonyms: cell-mediated immunity, delayed reaction.

DAN protocol: Defeat Autism Now! which comprises a network of doctors whose goal is to educate parents and clinicians about biomedically based research, appropriate testing, and safe and effective interventions for autism.

dopamine: A monoamine neurotransmitter that is formed during the synthesis of norepinephrine and is essential to the normal functioning of the central nervous system. A reduction of dopamine in the brain is associated with the development of Parkinson's disease. Chemical formula: $C8H11N02$.

dopaminergic: Of, relating to, or activated by dopamine or related substances.

erythromycins: A crystalline antibiotic produced by *Streptomyces erythreus* and used in the treatment of gram-positive bacterial infections. Erythromycin is most effective against gram-positive bacteria such as pneumococci, streptococci, and some staphylococci. The antibiotic also has some effect on gram-negative bacteria and some fungi. Erythromycin inhibits protein synthesis in susceptible microorganisms. It is used to treat such diseases as pneumonia caused by fungi, and streptococcus and syphilis infections, especially where the patient is allergic to penicillin.

fibromyalgia: Fibromyalgia is described as inflammation of the fibrous or connective tissue of the body. Widespread muscle pain, fatigue, and multiple tender points characterize these conditions. Fibrositis, fibromyalgia, and fibromyositis are names given to a set of symptoms believed to be caused by the same general problem.

frontal lobe: The frontal lobe is an area in the brain of mammals. Located at the front of each cerebral hemisphere, frontal lobes are positioned in front of (anterior to) the parietal lobes.

glial cells: Of or relating to neuroglia.

granule cells: Tiny neurons (a type of cell) that are around ten micrometers in diameter. Granule cells are found within the granular layer of the cerebellum.

HBOT: Hyperbaric oxygen therapy.

Herxheimer reaction: The Herxheimer reaction (also known as Jarisch-Herxheimer or herx) occurs when large quantities of toxins are released into the body as bacteria (typically spirochetal bacteria) die, due to antibiotic treatment. Typically the death of these bacteria and the associated release of endotoxins occurs faster than the body can remove the toxins via the natural detoxification process performed by the kidneys and liver. It is manifested by fever, chills, headache, myalgias, and exacerbation of cutaneous lesions. Duration in syphilis is normally only a few hours but can be much longer in other diseases. The intensity of the reaction reflects the intensity of inflammation present. The Herxheimer reaction has shown an increase in inflammatory cytokines during the period of exacerbation.

idiopathic: Relating to or being a disease having no known cause.

interleukins: A generic term for a group of multifunctional cytokines that are produced by a variety of lymphoid and nonlymphoid cells and whose effects occur at least partly within the lymphopoietic system.

Landau-Kleffner: LKS, also called infantile acquired aphasia, acquired epileptic aphasia or aphasia with convulsive disorder, is a rare, childhood neurological syndrome characterized by the sudden or gradual development of aphasia (the inability to understand or express language) and an abnormal electroencephalogram (EEG). LKS affects the parts of the brain that control comprehension and speech. The disorder usually occurs in children between the ages of five and seven years. Typically, children with LKS develop normally but then lose their language skills. While many of the affected individuals have clinical seizures, some only have electrographic seizures, including electrographic status epilepticus of sleep (ESES).

limbic system: Is a term for a set of brain structures including the hippocampus and amygdala and anterior thalamic nuclei and a limbic cortex that support a variety of functions including emotion, behavior, and long-term memory. The structures of the brain described by the limbic system are closely associated with the olfactory structures. The term "limbic" comes from Latin *limbus*, meaning "border" or "edge."

macrophages: "Big eaters," from makros "large" + phagein "eat") are cells within the tissues that originate from specific white blood cells called monocytes. Monocytes and macrophages are phagocytes, acting in both nonspecific defense (or innate immunity) as well as specific defense (or cell-mediated immunity) of vertebrate animals. Their role is to phagocytose (engulf and then digest) cellular debris and pathogens either as stationary or mobile cells, and to stimulate lymphocytes and other immune cells to respond to the pathogen.

magnetic resonance imaging (MRI): Uses magnetic fields and radio waves to produce high quality two- or three-dimensional images of brain structures without use of ionizing radiation (X-rays) or radioactive tracers. During an MRI, a large cylindrical magnet creates a magnetic field around the head of the patient through which radio waves are sent. When the magnetic field is imposed, each point in space has a unique radio frequency at which the signal is received and transmitted (Preuss). Sensors read the frequencies, and a computer uses the information to construct an image. The detection mechanisms are so precise that changes in structures over time can be detected. Using MRI, scientists can create images of both surface and subsurface structures with a high degree of anatomical detail. MRI scans can produce cross-sectional images in any direction from top to bottom, side to side, or front to back. The problem with original MRI technology was that while it provides a detailed assessment of the physical appearance, water content, and many kinds of subtle derangements of structure of the brain (such as inflammation or bleeding), it fails to provide information about the metabolism of the brain (how actively it is functioning) at the time of imaging. A distinction is therefore made between "MRI imaging" and "functional MRI imaging" (fMRI), where MRI provides only structural information on the brain while fMRI yields both structural and functional data.

multiple sclerosis (MS): A chronic autoimmune disorder affecting movement, sensation, and bodily functions. It is caused by destruction of the myelin insulation covering nerve fibers (neurons) in the central nervous system (brain and spinal cord).

neuronal loss: Loss of neurons (also known as neurones and nerve cells), which are electrically excitable cells in the nervous system that process and transmit information.

neurons (also known as neurones and nerve cells): Electrically excitable cells in the nervous system that process and transmit information. In vertebrate animals, neurons are the core components of the brain, spinal cord, and peripheral nerves.

NIDS: Neuro immune dysfunction syndromes, a set of related disorders characterized by complex interactions between the nervous system and the immune system.

norepinephrine: A hormone secreted by the adrenal medulla that is released into the bloodstream in response to physical or mental stress, as from fear or injury. It initiates many bodily responses, including the stimulation of heart action and an increase in blood pressure, metabolic rate, and blood glucose concentration. Also called adrenaline.

PANDAS: An abbreviation for Pediatric Autoimmune Neuropsychiatric Disorders Associated with Streptococcal infections.

pathophysiology: The study of the biologic and physical manifestations of disease as they correlate with the underlying abnormalities and physiologic disturbances. Pathophysiology does not deal directly with the treatment of disease. Rather, it explains the processes within the body that result in the signs and symptoms of a disease.

PET scan: Positron–emission tomography (PET) measures emissions from radioactively labeled metabolically active chemicals that have been injected into the bloodstream. The emission data are computer-processed to produce two- or three-dimensional images of the distribution of the chemicals throughout the brain (Nilsson 57). The positron-emitting radioisotopes used are produced by a cyclotron, and chemicals are labelled with these radioactive atoms. The labeled compound, called a radiotracer, is injected into the bloodstream and eventually makes its way to the brain. Sensors in the PET scanner detect the radioactivity as the compound accumulates in various regions of the brain. A computer uses the data gathered by the sensors to create multicolored two- or three-dimensional images that show where the compound acts in the brain. Especially useful are a wide array of ligands used to map different aspects of neurotransmitter activity, with by far the most commonly used PET tracer being a labeled form of glucose (see FDG).

Purkinje cells: A class of GABAergic neurons located in the cerebellar cortex. They are named after their discoverer, Czech anatomist Jan Evangelista Purkyně.

retroviruses: A retrovirus is an RNA virus that is replicated in a host cell via the enzyme reverse transcriptase to produce DNA from its RNA genome. The DNA is then incorporated into the host's genome by an integrase enzyme. The virus thereafter replicates as part of the host cell's DNA. They are enveloped viruses possessing an RNA genome, and replicate via a DNA intermediate.

RhoGam injections: A medicine given by intermuscular injection that is used to prevent the immunological condition known as Rhesus disease (or hemolytic disease of newborn). It can prevent maternal sensitization by Rh D antigens on the surface of blood cells from a Rhesus positive fetus in a Rhesus negative mother. The medicine is a solution of IgG anti-D (anti-RhD) antibodies which binds and destroys fetal Rh D positive red blood cells that have passed through the placenta from the fetus to the maternal circulation. This prevents maternal B-cell activation and memory cell formation. With the widespread use Rho(D) immune globulin Rh disease of the fetus and newborn has almost disappeared.

SPECT: Single photon emission computed tomography (SPECT) is similar to PET and uses gamma ray emitting radioisotopes and a gamma camera to record data that a computer uses to construct two- or three-dimensional images of active brain regions (ball). SPECT relies on an injection of radioactive tracer, which is rapidly taken up by the brain but does not redistribute. Uptake of SPECT agent is nearly 100 percent complete within 30—60s, reflecting cerebral blood flow (CBF) at the time of injection. These properties of SPECT make it particularly well suited for epilepsy imaging, which is usually made difficult by problems with patient movement and variable seizure types. SPECT provides a "snapshot" of cerebral blood flow since scans can be acquired after seizure termination (so long as the radioactive tracer was injected at the time of the seizure). A significant limitation of SPECT is its poor resolution (about 1 cm) compared to that of MRI.

temporal lobes: The temporal lobes are parts of the cerebrum that are involved in speech, memory, and hearing. They lie at the sides of the brain, beneath the lateral or Sylvian fissure.

thimerosal: A mercury-based crystalline powder with antibacterial and antifungal properties, used as a local antiseptic and preservative in vaccines and other drugs.

Tourette's: Tourette's syndrome (TS) is an inherited disorder of the nervous system, characterized by a variable expression of unwanted movements and noises (tics).

virus: a minute infectious agent which, with certain exceptions, is not resolved by the light microscope, lacks independent metabolism and is able to replicate only within a living host cell; the individual particle (virion) consists of nucleic acid (nucleoid)—DNA or RNA (but not both)—and a protein shell (capsid), which contains and protects the nucleic acid and which may be multilayered.

NOTES

Foreword

1. Goldstein, J. The Pathophysiology and Treatment of Chronic Fatigue Syndrome and Other Neurosomatic Disorders: Cognitive Therapy in a Pill. Alasbimn Journal2(7): April 2000. Article N° AJ07-5. http://www.alasbimnjournal.cl/revistas/7/goldstein.html
2. Goldberg, M. Mena I and Miller B. Frontal and Temporal Lobe Dysfunction in autism and Other Related Disorders: ADHD and OCD. Alasbimn Journal1(4): July 1999. http://www.alasbimnjournal.cl/revistas/4/goldberg.htm
3. Roca Bielsa, I. ; Mena, I.; García-Burillo, A. et al. SPET cerebral cuantificado en el Síndrome de Fatiga Crónica: comparación de los estudios basal y post-esfuerzo. Alasbimn Journal 8(31): January 2006.
4. Mena G., Ismael. Neurospect applications in Psychiatry. Alasbimn Journal 11 (45):July 2009. Article N° AJ45-1.http://www.alasbimnjournal.cl/
5. Mountz J., Tolbert L., Lill D., Katholi C., and Liu H. Functional Deficit in Autistic Disorder< Characterization by Tc99m HMPAO and SPECT. J.Nuc.Med.1995, 36, 1156/1162

Introduction

Klotter, Jule. (2002) Hepatitis B Vaccine TownsendLetter (In the case of the hepatitis B vaccine, Samuel L. Katz, MD, who was ACIP chairman when the hepatitis B recommendations were made in 1991, admitted that no peer-reviewed, published studies supported giving the vaccine to newborns. Mr . Belkin says that over . . . In the case of the hepatitis B vaccine, Samuel L. Katz, MD, who was ACIP chairman when the hepatitis B recommendations were made in 1991, admitted that no peer-reviewed, published studies supported giving the vaccine to newborns. Mr . Belkin says that over 36,000 adverse reactions and 440 deaths involving the hepatitis B vaccine have been reported to the Vaccine Adverse Event Reporting System.)

Chapter 4

1. Delong, G. R., S. C. Bean, and F. R. Brown III. (1981) Acquired reversible autistic syndrome in acute encephalopathic illness in children. *Archives of Neurology* 38: 191,194.

2. Gillberg, C. (1986). Brief report: Onset at age 14 of a typical autistic syndrome. A case report of a girl with herpes simplex encephalitis. *Journal of Autism and Developmental Disorders* 16: 369–375.

3. Greer, M. K., M. Lyons-Crews, L. B. Mauldin, and F. R. Brown III. (1989) A case study of the cognitive and behavioral deficits of temporal lobe damage in herpes simplex encephalitis. *Journal of Autism and Developmental Disorders* 19: 317–326.

4. Plioplys, A. V., A. Greaves, W. Yoshida. (1989) Anti-CNS antibodies in childhood neurologic diseases. *Neuropediatrics* 20: 93–102.

5. Boucher, J., and E. K. Warrington. (1976) Memory deficits in early infantile autism: Some similarities to the amnesic syndrome. *British Journal of Psychology* 67: 76–87.

6. Hauser, S. L., G. R. DeLong, N. P. Rosman (1975) Pneumographic findings in the infantile autism syndrome: A correlation with temporal lobe disease. *Brain* 98: 667–688.

7. Damasio, A.R., and R. G. Maurer. (1978) A neurological model for childhood autism. *Archives of Neurology* 35: 777–789.

8. Courchesne, E. (1991) Neuroanatomic imaging in autism. *Pediatrics* 87: 781–890.

9. (Ref: 1981 DeLong, 1986; Gillberg, 1989). Delong, G. R., S. C. Bean, and F. R. Brown III. (1981) Acquired reversible autistic syndrome in acute encephalopathic illness in children. *Archives of Neurology* 38: 191,194.

   Gillberg, C. (1986). Brief report: Onset at age 14 of a typical autistic syndrome. A case report of a girl with herpes simplex encephalitis. *Journal of Autism and Developmental Disorders* 16: 369–375.

   Greer, M. K., M. Lyons-Crews, L. B. Mauldin, and F. R. Brown III. (1989) A case study of the cognitive and behavioral deficits of temporal lobe damage in herpes simplex encephalitis. *Journal of Autism and Developmental Disorders* 19: 317–326.

10. Jay, V., et al. (1995) Pathology of chronic herpes infection associated with seizure disorder. *Pediatric Pathology and Labroatory Medicine* 15: 131–146.

11. Sanders, V. J., et al. (1997) Presence of herpes simplex DNA in surgical tissue from human epileptic seizure foci detected by polymerase chain reaction. *Archives of Neurology* 54: 9554–9560.

12. Marlowe, W. B., E. L. Namcall, and J. J. Thomas. (1975) Complete Klüver-Bucy syndrome in man. *Cortex* 11, 53–59.

13. Behan, P. O., W. M. H. Behan, and E. J. Bell. (1985) The post-viral fatigue syndrome. *Journal of Infectious Diseases* 10: 211–222.

14. Borysiewicz, L. K., S. J. Haworth, J. Cohen, J. Mundin, A. Rickinson, and J. G. P. Sissons. (1986) Epstein-Barr virus-specific immune defects in patients with persistent symptoms following infectious mononucleosis. *QJM* 58: 111–21

15. Jones, J. F., C. G. Ray, L. L. Minnich, M. J. Hicks, R. Kibler, D. O. Locas. (1985) Evidence of active Epstein-Barr virus infection in patients with persistant, unexplained illnesses: elevated anti-early antigen antigen antibodies. *Annals of Internal Medicine* 102: 1–7.

16. Kroenke, K., D. R. Wood, A. D. Mangelsdorff, N. J. Meier, and J. B. Powell. (1988) Chronic fatigue in primary care: prevalence, patient characteristics, and outcome. *JAMA* 260: 929–934.

17. Holmes, G. P., J. E. Kaplan, J. A. Stewart, B. Hunt, P. F. Pinsky, L. B. Schonberger. (1987) A cluster of patients with a chronic mononucleosis-like syndrome: is Epstein-Barr virus the cause? *JAMA* 257: 2297–2302.

18. Krueger, G. R. F., B. Koch, D. V. Albashi. (1987) Persistent fatigue and depression in patients with anti-body to human B-lymphotropic virus. *Lancet* 2: 36.

19. Jenkins, R. (1991) Post-viral fatigue syndrome. Epidemiology: lessons from the past. *British Medical Bulletin* 47(4): 952–965.

20. Wallace, P. G. (1991) Post-viral fatigue syndrome. Epidemiology: a critical review. *British Medical Bulletin* 47 (4) : 942–951.

21. O'Meara, M., et al. (1996) Viral encephalitis in children. *Current Opinion in Pediatrics* 8: 11–15.

22. Hetzler, B., and J. Griffin. (1981) Infantile autism and the temporal lobe of the brain. *Journal of Autism and Developmental Disorders* 11: 317–330.

23. Jones, P. B., and R. W. Kerwin. (1990) Left temporal lobe damage in Asperger's syndrome. *British Journal of Psychiatry* 156: 570–572.

24. Courchesne, E. (1991) Neuro-anatomic imaging in autism. *Pediatrics* 87: 781–890.

25. Greer, M. K., M. Lyons-Crews, L. B. Mauldin, and F. R. Brown III. (1989) A case study of the cognitive and behavioral deficits of temporal lobe damage in herpes simplex encephalitis. *Journal of Autism and Developmental Disorders* 19: 317–326.

26. Ghaziuddin, M., L. Y. Tsai, L. Eilers, and N. Ghaziuddin. (1992) Brief Report: Autism and Herpes Simplex Encephalitis. *Journal of Autism and Developmental Disorders* 22 (1).

27. Boucher J., and E. K. Warrington. (1976) Memory deficits in early infantile autism: Some similarities to the amnesic syndrome. *British Journal of Psychology*. 76–87.

28. Hauser S. L., G. R. DeLong, and N. P. Rosman. (1975) Pneumographic findings in the infantile autism syndrome: A correlation with temporal lobe disease. *Brain* 98: 667–688.

29. Hetzler, B., and J. Griffin, J. (1981) Infantile autism and the temporal lobe of the brain. *Journal of Autism and Developmental Disorders* 11: 317–330.

30. Jones, P. B., and R. W. Kerwin (1990). Left temporal lobe damage in Asperger's syndrome. *British Journal of Psychiatry*, 156, 570–572.

Chapter 5

1. Plioplys, A. V. (1994) Autism: EEG abnormalities and clinical improvement with valproic acid. *Archives of Pediatrics & Adolescent Medicine* 148: 220–222

2. Ichise, M., I. E. Salit, S. E. Abbey, D. G. Chung, B. Gray, J. C. Kirsh, and M. Freedman. (1992) Assessment of regional cerebral perfusion in 99 Tem-HMPAO SPECT in chronic fatigue syndrome. *Nuclear Medicine Communications* 13: 767–772.

3. Costa D. C., J. Brostoff, and P. J. Ell. (1992) Brain stem hypoperfusion in patients with myalgic encephalomyelitis- chronic fatigue syndrome (abstract) *European Journal of Nuclear Medicine* 19(8): 733.

4. Weizman, A., R. Weizman, G. A. Szekely, H. Wijsenbeek, and E. Livni. (1982) Abnormal immune response to brain tissue antigen in the syndrome of autism. *American Journal of Psychiatry* 7: 1462–1465.

5. Todd, R. D., and R. D. Ciaranello. (1985) Demonstration of inter- and intraspecies differences in serotonin binding sites by antibodies from an autistic child. *PNAS* 82: 612–616.

6. Singh, V. K., H. H. Fudenberg, D. Emerson, and M. Coleman. (1988) Immunodiagnosis and immunotherapy in autistic children. *Annals of the New York Academy of Sciences* 540: 602–604.

7. Plioplys, A. V. (1989) Autism: immunologic investigations, in Gillberg, C. (ed): *Diagnosis and Treatment of Autism*. New York: Plenum, pp. 133–138.

8. Plioplys, A. V. (1994) Selective suppression of maternal IgG anti-central nervous system antibody reactivity. *Developmental Brain Dysfunction* 7:165–170.

9. Funderburk, S. J., J. Carter, P. Tanguay, B. J. Freeman, and J. R. Westlake. (1983) Parental reproductive problems and gestational hormone exposure in autistic and schizophrenic children. *Journal of Autism and Developmental Disorders* 13: 325–332.

10. Stubbs, E. G., E. R. Ritvo, and A. Mason-Brothers. (1985) Autism and shared paternal HLA antigens. *Journal of the American Academy of Child and Adolescent Psychiatry* 24: 182–185.

11. Peterson, M. R., and E. F. Torrey. (1976) Viruses and other infectious agents as behavioral teratogens. In: *The Autistic Syndrome*, ed. M. Coleman. (New York: American Elsevier.)

12. Warren, R. P., P. Cole, D. Odell, et al. (1990) Detection of maternal antibodies in Infantile Autism. *Journal of the American Academy of Child and Adolescent Psychiatry* 29 (6): 873–877.

13. McConnachie, P. R., and J. A. McIntyre. (1984) Maternal antipaternal immunity in couples predisposed to repeated pregnancy losses. *AJRIM* 5: 145–150.

14. Faulk, W. P., and J. A. McIntyre. (1981), Trophoblast survival. *Transplantation* 31: 1–5.

15. McIntyre, A., and W. P. Faulk. (1982) Allotypic trophoblast-lymphocyte cross reactive cell surface antigens. *Human Immunology* 4: 27–36.

16. Plioplys, A. V., A. Greaves, K. Kazemi, and E. Silverman. (1994) Lymphocyte function in autism and Rett syndrome. *Neuropsychobiology* 29: 12–16.

17. Yonk, L. J., R. P. Warren, R. A. Burger, P. Cole, J. D. Odell, W. L. Warren, E. White, and V. K. Singh. (1990) CD4+ helper T cell depression in autism. *Immunology Letters* 25: 341–346.

18. Warren, R. P., L. J. Yonk, R. A. Burger, P. Cole, J. D. Odell, W. L. Warren, E. White, E., and V. K. Singh. (1990) Deficiency of suppressor-induced (CD4+CD45RA+) T cells in autism. *Immunological Investigations* 19: 245–251.

19. Warren, R. P., V. K. Singh, P. Cole, J. D. Ode, C. B. Pincer, W. L. Warren, and E. White, E. (1991) Increased frequency of the null allele at the complement C4b locus in autism. *Clinical & Experimental Immunology* 83: 438–440.

20. Morimoto, C., E. L. Rheinherz, S. F. Schlossman, P. H. Schur, J. A. Mills, and A. D. Steinberg. (1980) Alterations in immunoregulatory T cell subsets in active systemic lupus erthematosus, *Journal of Clinical Investigation* 66: 1171–1174.

21. Morimoto, C., D. A. Hafler, H. L. Weiner, N. L. Letvin, M. Hagan, J. Daley, and S. F. Schlossman. (1987) Selective loss of the suppressor-inducer T cell subset in progressive

multiple sclerosis: Analysis with anti-2H4 monoclonal antibody. *New England Journal of Medicine* 316: 67–72.

22. Plioplys, A. V., A. Greaves, K. Kazemi, and E. Silverman. (1994) Lymphocyte function in autism and Rett syndrome. *Neuropsychobiology* 29: 12–16.

23. Plioplys, A.V., A. Greaves, K. Kazemi, E. Silverman. (1994) Immunologic reactivity in autism and Rett syndrome. *Developmental Brain Dysfunction* 7:12–16.

24. Toh, G. H., et al. (1985) Proceedings of the National Academy of Sciences 82: 3485.

25. Galbraith, G. M. P., et al. (1986) The Journal of Clinical Investigation 78: 865.

26. Toh, G. H., et al. (1985) Proceedings of the National Academy of Sciences 82: 3485.

27. Plioplys, A.V., Greaves, A. Kazemi, K., Silverman, E. Immunologic reactivity in autism and Rett syndrome. Developmental Brain Dysfunction. 7:12-16, 1994

28. Plioplys, A. V. (1999) Treatment of autistic children with intravenous immunoglobulin. *Journal of Child Neurology* 14: 203–205.

29. Singh V. K., R. P. Warren, J. D. Ode, and P. Cole. (1991) Changes of soluble interleukin-2, interleukin-2 receptor, T8 antigen, and interleukin-1 in the serum of autistic children. *Clinical Immunology and Immunopathology* 61: 448–455.

30. Chess, S. (1971) Autism in children with congenital rubella. *Journal of Autism & Childhood Schizophrenia* 1: 33–47.

31. Stubbs, E. G., E. Ash, and P. S. Williams. (1983) Autism and congenital cytomegalovirus. *Journal of Autism and Developmental Disorders* 14: 249–253.

32. Goldberg, M. J., I. Mena, and J. Darcourt J. (1997) NeuroSPECT findings in children with chronic fatigue syndrome. *Journal of Chronic Fatigue Syndrome* 3 (1): 61–67.

33. Weizman, A. , Weizman, R., Szekely, G.A., Wijsenbeek, H., and Livni, E. , Abnormal immune response to brain tissue antigen in the syndrome of autism, Am. J. Psychiatry 7, 1462-1465, 1982

    35Todd, R.D., and Ciaranello, R.D., Demonstration of inter- and intraspecies differences in serotonin binding sites by antibodies from an autistic child, Proc. Natl. Acad. Sci. USA 82, 612-616,1985

    Singh, V.K., Fudenberg, H.H., Emerson, D. and Coleman, M., Immunodiagnosis and immunotherapy in autistic children, Ann. N. Y. Acad. Sci. 540, 602-604, 1988

    Plioplys, A.V.: Autism: immunologic investigations, in Gillberg, C. (ed): Diagnosis and Treatment of Autism, New York, Plenum Press, pp. 133-138, 1989.

Plioplys, A.V. Selective suppression of maternal IgG anti-central nervous system antibody reactivity. Developmental Brain Dysfunction. 7:165-170, 1994.

34. Immunological Findings in Autism. (2005) *International Review of Neurobiology*71: 317–341.

35. Riazi, K., M. A. Galic, J. B. Kuzmiski, W. Ho, and K. A. Sharkey. (November 4, 2008) Microglial activation and TNFalpha production mediate altered CNS excitability following peripheral inflammation *Pittman Proceedings of the National Academy of Sciences of the United States of America*105 (44): 17151–17156.

36. Michael Goldberg, Ismael Mena, and Bruce Miller. (July 1999) Frontal and temporal lobe dysfunction in autism other related disorders: ADHD and OCD. *Alasbimn Journal* 1(4).

Chapter 7

1. Ashman, R. B., J. M. Papadimitrious, A.K. Ott, et al. (1990) Antigens and immune responses in *Candida albicans* infection. *Immunology & Cell Biology* 68: 1–13.
Wilton, J. M. A., and T. Lehner, T. (1980) Immunology of candidiasis.
Developmental and Comparative Immunology 8: 525–559.

2. Syverson, R. E., H. Buckley, J. Gibian, et al. (1979) Cellular and humoral immune status in women with chronic Candida vaginitis. *American Journal of Obstetrics & Gynecology*143: 624–627.

3. Witkin, S. S., M. S. Ing Ru, and W. J. Ledger. (1983) Inhibition of *Candida albicans*–induced lymphocyte proliferation by lymphocytes and sera from women with recurrent vaginitis. *American Journal of Obstetrics & Gynecology* 147: 809–811.

4. Kirkpatrick, C. H. (1988) Chronic mucocutaneous candidiasis. Antibiotic and immunologic therapy. *Annals of the New York Academy of Sciences* 544: 471–480.

5. Swedo SE, Leonard HL, Garvey M, Mittleman B, Allen AJ, Perlmutter S, Lougee L, Dow S, Zamkoff J, Dubbert BK. (1998) Pediatric autoimmune neuropsychiatric disorders associated with streptococcal infections: clinical description of the first 50 cases.
The American Journal of Psychiatry 155(2):264-71. Erratum in: *The American Journal of Psychiatry* 1998 Apr;155(4):578.

6. Perlmutter SJ, Garvey MA, Castellanos X, Mittleman BB, Giedd J, Rapoport JL, Swedo SE. (1998) A case of pediatric autoimmune neuropsychiatric disorders associated with

streptococcal infections. *The American Journal of Psychiatry* 155(11):1592-8. No abstract available.

7. Swedo SE, Leonard HL, Mittleman BB, Allen AJ, Rapoport JL, Dow SP, Kanter ME, Chapman F, Zabriskie J. (1997) Identification of children with pediatric autoimmune neuropsychiatric disorders associated with streptococcal infections by a marker associated with rheumatic fever. *The American Journal of Psychiatry* 154(1):110-2.

8. Swedo SE, Garvey M, Snider L, Hamilton C, Leonard HL. (2001) The PANDAS subgroup: recognition and treatment.
    CNS Spectrums 6(5):419-22, 425-6.

9. Einarson A. (2010) Paroxetine use in pregnancy and increased risk of heart defects: Evaluating the evidence. *Canadian Family Physician* 56(8):767-8.

10. Tuccori M, Montagnani S, Testi A, Ruggiero E, Mantarro S, Scollo C, Pergola A, Fornai M, Antonioli L, Colucci R, Corona T, Blandizzi C. (2010) Use of selective serotonin reuptake inhibitors during pregnancy and risk of major and cardiovascular malformations: an update. *Postgraduate Medicine* 122(4):49-65.

11. Ellfolk M, Malm H. (2010) Risks associated with in utero and lactation exposure to selective serotonin reuptake inhibitors (SSRIs). *Reproductive Toxicology* Sep;30(2):249-60. Epub 2010 May 4.

Chapter 8

1. A joint statement of the American Academy of Family Physicians (AAFP), The American Academy Of Pediatrics (AAP), The Advisory Committee On Immunization Practices (ACIP), and The United States Public Health Service (PHS) http://www.aap.org/policy/JOINTthim.html.

Chapter 11

1. Kelly, A., and K. Khan. (2008) Prevalence of allergies in children with complex medical problems. *Clinical Pediatrics* 47(8): 809–816.